4

Finally, a book worth recommending to women coping with the loss of a pregnancy. Wenzel uses her expert knowledge of cognitive behavioral therapy techniques, along with her own firsthand experience, to produce a clear and powerful guide that will help you through this difficult period. The many forms and worksheets make this a very user-friendly resource.

—**Jonathan S. Abramowitz, PhD,** Professor and Associate Chair of Psychology, University of North Carolina at Chapel Hill

Thoroughly grounded in evidence-based research, this is a rich compendium of tools for those who have experienced the heartbreak of a pregnancy loss or infertility. It "speaks" in the sensitive and compassionate voice of Dr. Wenzel, who herself experienced reproductive loss. This book validates your grief and provides specific ideas to help you heal and grow, find meaning, and cultivate strength and wisdom. The resultant coping skills will guide you for the rest of your life.

—**Joann Paley Galst, PhD,** private practice, Women's Mental Health Consortium, New York, NY

As I read this book, I found myself applying Wenzel's wise words to the experiences of my clients as well as to my own experience. Although I am sorry you have a reason to be reading this book, I am very glad you have found it. It will walk you through the process of finding hope and healing.

—**Keri Kitchen, MEd, LPCC, NCC,** founder of the Carys Rainn Foundation, Grayson, KY

Coping With Infertility, Miscarriage, and Neonatal Loss

Coping With Infertility, Miscarriage, and Neonatal Loss

Finding Perspective and Creating Meaning

AMY WENZEL, PhD

American Psychological Association • Washington, DC

Published by
APA LifeTools
750 First Street, NE
Washington, DC 20002
www.apa.org

To order
APA Order Department
P.O. Box 92984
Washington, DC 20090-2984
Tel: (800) 374-2721;
Direct: (202) 336-5510
Fax: (202) 336-5502;
TDD/TTY: (202) 336-6123
Online: www.apa.org/pubs/books
E-mail: order@apa.org

In the U.K., Europe, Africa, and the Middle East, copies may be ordered from
American Psychological Association
3 Henrietta Street
Covent Garden, London
WC2E 8LU England

Typeset in Sabon by Circle Graphics, Inc., Columbia, MD

Printer: Edwards Brothers, Inc., Ann Arbor, MI
Cover Designer: Naylor Design, Washington, DC

The opinions and statements published are the responsibility of the authors, and such opinions and statements do not necessarily represent the policies of the American Psychological Association.

Library of Congress Cataloging-in-Publication Data
Wenzel, Amy, author.
  Coping with infertility, miscarriage, and neonatal loss : finding perspective and creating meaning / Amy Wenzel.
    pages cm
  Includes bibliographical references and index.
  ISBN 978-1-4338-1692-5 — ISBN 1-4338-1692-X 1. Infertility—Psychological aspects. 2. Miscarriage—Psychological aspects. 3. Perinatal death—Psychological aspects. 4. Stillbirth—Psychological aspects. I. Title.
  RC889.W393 2014
  618.3'9—dc23
                                    2013039238

British Library Cataloguing-in-Publication Data
A CIP record is available from the British Library.

Printed in the United States of America
First Edition

http://dx.doi.org/10.1037/14391-000

To my unborn babies.
May your legacy live on.

CONTENTS

ACKNOWLEDGMENTS

I give my heartfelt thanks to the LifeTools Division of APA Books for allowing me to compile this important and personally meaningful book. In particular, I appreciate the patience of Maureen Adams, who gave me the freedom and space to pull together my professional and personal experience into the final product. Although it was hard, at times, to write this book, it is my sincerest wish that it resonates with women and men who have experienced one or more reproductive losses.

Coping With Infertility, Miscarriage, and Neonatal Loss

INTRODUCTION

Perhaps the most dreaded nightmare for adults of childbearing age is a pregnancy loss. Pregnancy loss can create profound feelings of despair in expectant parents regardless of whether the loss occurs earlier in pregnancy (i.e., miscarriage), later in pregnancy (i.e., neonatal loss), or in the short period of time after a baby is born. In many instances, the same set of emotions occurs when a couple learns that their fertility treatments were unsuccessful. Drs. Janet Jaffe and Martha Diamond, two expert psychologists who specialize in perinatal psychology, referred to this collective grouping of reproductive events as *reproductive trauma*. I also refer to this collective grouping of events as *reproductive loss* because in all instances one experiences the loss of a greatly anticipated addition to the family that was expected to add a layer of meaning in life, perhaps like no other event could do. Throughout the book, I use the terms *reproductive loss*, *pregnancy loss*, and *reproductive trauma* interchangeably.

Many people who have experienced reproductive loss observe that there are few established rituals in today's society for grieving such events, in contrast to the rituals for grieving the loss of a parent, spouse, or a close family member. They find that however well-intentioned a sympathetic comment or word of comfort, it usually seems like the wrong thing. Furthermore, they are bombarded by constant media reports of celebrities who recently gave birth, who are pregnant, and who are expanding their families through expensive means that most people can only dream about. When they go grocery shopping, it seems like everyone else in the store is pushing an adorable little baby or toddler in the shopping cart. In the meantime, they are left to cope with an excruciating sense of emptiness.

I know, because I've been there. As a clinical psychologist who specializes in perinatal psychology, I have worked with countless women who have experienced pregnancy losses and other reproductive traumas. More important for the purpose of this book, I experienced my own series of reproductive losses: At 21 weeks' gestation into my first pregnancy at age 37, I lost my son due to premature rupture of membranes; on another occasion, I was "technically" pregnant for a week or so, but my human chorionic gonadotropin levels didn't rise like they should have; and I went through time-consuming and unsuccessful fertility treatments.

How does one cope with these excruciatingly difficult life events? Therapy is certainly an option and can provide a great deal of comfort; however, I do not want to imply that there is something pathological about grieving the loss of an unborn child and that professional intervention is absolutely essential. In fact, I would caution people who have experienced reproductive loss to choose their therapist carefully, as professional training in a mental health discipline does not guarantee that the provider possesses the knowledge and sensitivity needed to work with the fallout from this life event. Another option to which people who have experienced reproductive loss often turn is books that they expect will help them to understand their emotions, normalize their experiences, and feel a part of a broader community of people who have experienced similar losses.

Unfortunately, my own experience and the experiences of many of my clients were that reading many of the books on the market, quite simply, made us feel *worse*. It's not that these books lacked sensitivity and compassion—without fail, they were exquisitely sensitive and compassionate. The issue was that although we expected to gain comfort from stories of people who had also experienced a reproductive loss, it turned out that the last thing we needed was to read tearjerkers about a subject so close to home. In addition, we inevitably compared ourselves to the people described in these books. If a woman highlighted in a case description experienced multiple pregnancy losses, those of us who experienced only one loss would ruminate over the likelihood that we would have another one, concluding that it was certain that we would experience a subsequent loss. If a woman highlighted in a case description experienced a loss subsequent to having a healthy baby, those of us who had no children found ourselves feeling resentful and wondering how this situation could possibly apply to us—at least this woman *had* a child. Even when a case description matched up remarkably well to our own circumstances, we could always find nuances that made us view our own situations as far more hopeless and tenuous than theirs (e.g., "Yes, but I'm over 40, and she was only 35").

Moreover, the focus on case descriptions in many of these books left little room for discussion of actual strategies for coping with and healing from the loss. I and others had similar reactions—"Just tell us what to do! Just tell us how we can begin to make sense of this, work through this, and, though we might not be the same again, develop a sense of clarity, peace, and optimism for the future." We realized that there is no one-size-fits-all approach, but we wanted *something*.

In my own situation, I found that my training in evidence-based approaches to psychotherapy, particularly cognitive behavioral therapy (CBT), was a tremendous asset in helping me cope with my loss and my uncertainty about the future. The basic premise underlying CBT is that the meanings that we attribute to our life experiences, as well as the behaviors in which we engage in order to cope and live a quality life, have a profound effect on our mood. These attributions and behaviors also influence the likelihood of developing or experiencing a recurrence of a mood or anxiety disorder. In other words, how we think about the loss, and what we do about it, plays a large role in how we cope, achieve acceptance, and eventually adapt. Cognitive behavioral therapists use a number of active strategies to identify, evaluate, and modify unhelpful thoughts and attributions; strategies to engage in adaptive behaviors in the face of life stress; and strategies to attain acceptance and centeredness. My clients and I found that the gradual, empathetic, and compassionate application of these strategies gave us tangible skills for dealing with the loss that we could not find in most other books on the market. We found that applying these strategies in our daily lives helped us to break out of the cycle of sadness and rumination and gain perspective on and acceptance of the loss. As I was recovering from my second trimester loss, I continually reflected on my good fortune of being a cognitive behavioral therapist because I relied on the tried-and-true mood-management strategies on which I had been coaching my own clients for years. I honestly believe that I would have been paralyzed with grief, numbness, and lack of acceptance for a much longer period of time than I was without the active application of these strategies.

Thus, my purpose in contributing yet another book on reproductive loss to the market is to describe the specific tools that my clients and I have used to cope with pregnancy loss, infertility, and any other circumstances related to a reproductive loss or trauma. It addresses what I see as such a gap in the writing on this topic—how, *specifically*, does one cope, find perspective, create meaning, achieve acceptance, and take care of oneself after such a devastating event for which there exist few supports and resources? The tools described in this book have been evaluated by research examining cognitive behavioral treatment packages, which have been shown to be efficacious relative to not using any coping tools at all or to non-specific approaches to treatment such as supportive psychotherapy. Throughout the book, I describe specific ways to adapt these techniques on the basis of my own experience and my experience in helping my clients implement them in their lives.

Here's a snapshot of what you will learn in this book:

- In Chapter 1, you will learn about the grieving process. You will learn that it is OK to be feeling, thinking, and doing as you are even if others are strongly encouraging you to move on and even if the way you are feeling, thinking, and doing is very uncharacteristic of you.
- In Chapter 2, you will learn about tools that can help you get by in the first weeks following a reproductive loss. Some of these tools are not necessarily long-term solutions for helping you make decisions and enhance your quality of life, but they will help you survive the moments filled with pain and emptiness.
- In Chapter 3, you will learn about ways to reconnect and become actively engaged in your life in a meaningful, valued way, even when you don't feel like doing so. We know that active engagement in activities that are consistent with your values, strengths, and interests serves as a strong buffer against depression and other negative emotional experiences. Inactivity and isolation are more than understandable after a reproductive loss or trauma. But, after a period of time, they will unequivocally make things worse.
- In Chapter 4, you will learn how to cope with and manage disturbing thoughts and images of the pregnancy or unsuccessful infertility treatments and their immediate implications.

Specifically, you will learn to identify when these thoughts and images are activated, obtain some distance from them, and reevaluate them so that you are viewing these experiences in a balanced manner, as accurately and helpfully as possible. You will also be introduced to a strategy to address thoughts and images that you experience as intrusive. These thoughts and images do not have to hang over you like a black cloud or color the way you view other events in your life.

- In Chapter 5, you will apply the tools that you learned in Chapter 4 to cope with disturbing thoughts and images of the longer term future. You will also learn tools for accepting and coping with the uncertainty of your reproductive future. Difficulty coping with uncertainty is a key contributor to anxiety, apprehension, and stress, and developing this skill will help you to manage the curveballs that life throws for many years to come.

- In Chapter 6, you will learn tools for interacting with others in a variety of circumstances that are difficult after a reproductive loss. How do you share the news of the loss with other family members? How do you maintain a fulfilling relationship with a pregnant friend who seemed to have conceived so easily? How do you respond to well-meaning people who unintentionally make unhelpful or insensitive comments? How do you connect with a spouse or a partner who is handling the event much differently than you are? Chapter 6 addresses these and other circumstances.

- Chapter 7 was written for people who find themselves to be especially avoidant of reminders of their loss, such as situations in which they might encounter women who are pregnant or families who have small children. This chapter outlines a step-by-step procedure for overcoming this avoidance.

- In Chapter 8, you will learn tools that will help you to make sound, informed decisions about your reproductive future. You will also learn that it is OK to ultimately choose solutions that, on the surface, are associated with many disadvantages in order to achieve your most valued outcomes.
- In Chapter 9, you will learn tools for achieving a present-focused, nonjudgmental mind, a process called *mindfulness*. Mindfulness allows you to form a new relationship with your emotional pain, and even with any physical pain you might be experiencing, such that the pain becomes less adversarial and threatening. The practice of mindfulness helps people to accept their life circumstances and let go of struggles that they cannot change. This chapter will give you ideas for integrating mindfulness into the manner in which you live your life.
- In Chapter 10, you will work toward finding meaning from the tragedy of your reproductive loss. You will create what I like to call a *new normal*. This chapter will help you pull together the material and tools described throughout the book for you to gain wisdom and growth from your experience and to create a life well lived, regardless of your reproductive outcome.

The most important lesson that I've learned from my own and my clients' experiences is that every reproductive loss is different. Although the woman's age, the length of gestation, history of previous pregnancy losses, and the amount of time and money devoted to conceiving are important variables, the key is the *meaning* that the person attaches to the pregnancy. Generally speaking, the more psychological and emotional investment a person places in the pregnancy, the more difficult will be the experience of loss or trauma. This is coupled with the fact that we all have our own history and even "baggage," such as the early loss of one of our own parents, scars from past childhood sexual abuse, or the expectation that we could "have it all" and establish a career before embarking on family planning. All of these historical, psychological, emotional, and situational factors contribute to what Drs. Jaffe and Diamond referred to as the *reproductive story*, which is the vision that we have created about our transition to parenthood and subsequent family composition. The unique experience of a reproductive loss, then, is intricately tied to your reproductive story; reproductive loss disrupts your reproductive story and forces you to confront the possibility that your desired story will not be realized. This experience is different for everyone because everyone's reproductive loss and reproductive stories are unique.

What this means is that not all of the material covered in this book will be right for you. There might even be times that you think to yourself, "How can she be suggesting this? This will just make me feel worse." Keep in mind that you are the expert on your own tendencies, preferences, history, and reproductive story. And, all things being equal, I fully recognize that readers already know how to take care of themselves. The issue at hand, however, is that all things are *not* equal at the moment—the reader will have likely experienced a devastating reproductive loss or trauma, and many of her adaptive coping and self-care skills may have gone out the window. It is my hope that this book can serve as a concrete resource for people who have experienced reproductive loss to consult when they can't imagine, or can't remember, how to take care of themselves and make sense of their recent life events.

When you do identify one or more tools that might be a good match for you, my suggestion is to keep an open mind and systematically practice them for good chunk of time (i.e., a few weeks at least). I say this because learning most of these tools is akin to acquiring skills such as riding a bicycle. They are not perfected in one instance. In fact, people often find that when they first try to apply the tools during a time of acute emotional distress, they are disappointed that they do not feel better. The reason for this is that it is difficult to learn and perfect a tool in times of emotional distress—your attention is divided, your mind is elsewhere, and you are experiencing overwhelming emotions. Thus, it is often best to practice the tools in times of (relative) calm so that you develop skillfulness in their application and can later apply them to acute emotional distress.

I have a couple of caveats pertaining to things that I have deliberately chosen *not* to include in this book. The purpose of this book is not to be a comprehensive resource on understanding every facet of pregnancy loss or reproductive trauma. I provide few statistics because, although they might instill hope that people who have experienced reproductive loss are not alone, more often they also instill a great deal of fear and apprehension about future pregnancies. Rather, this book is meant to be a source of tangible suggestions for coping and building a meaningful life in the wake of the tragedy, providing wisdom, inspiration, and hope. It will not provide detailed steps on ways to handle every facet of postloss challenges, but it will give you a framework for gaining perspective and taking care of yourself.

In addition, although at times I illustrate the application of these cognitive behavioral tools using case examples, the details of the actual loss in each example are kept to a minimum. In most cases, I also do not include reference to the individual's age, whether the individual has other children, or whether the individual went on to have a successful pregnancy. Instead, the case examples focus on the manner in which people who have experienced reproductive loss use their strengths and resources in their lives to manage their grief, build meaning in their lives, and take care of themselves. Inclusion of details such as the individual's age, family composition, and ultimate reproductive outcome invariably facilitates unhelpful comparisons. This is just too hard for people who have no children and who are unsure of whether there is a child in their future, for people who have one child and who desperately want more but who are having trouble conceiving, and for people who have two or more children but who anticipate that they will feel unfulfilled until they have another child.

Before closing this Introduction, I'd like to say that this book is appropriate for both women and men. Too often, men's experiences of pregnancy loss and infertility, or even pregnancy in general, go unacknowledged. The reproductive story can be every bit as meaningful to men as it is to women. For this reason, in many instances, I refer to "people" and "individuals" rather than to "women" per se. At times, however, I was forced to include a pronoun, and in these instances I chose "she" to avoid clunkiness in the writing. However, I want my male readers to know that the material in most sentences that reference "she" can apply to them as well.

Woman or man, one does not necessarily "get over" a reproductive loss. It changes who you are; it alters your sense of safety, predictability, and even justice; and it reminds you that life is far from easy. But you *can* cope effectively, and with time, you will be able to achieve acceptance, create meaning from the experience, and take care of yourself. Even if your reproductive story ultimately turns out very differently from how you had hoped, you will be able to live your life according to your values and strengths and gain lasting fulfillment. This book describes many well-established strategies for doing so, tailored, of course, to the unique experience of reproductive loss. As time passes after the initial event, some days will be better than others. Your reaction to this book might even be different at different times. Sometimes you may find it hopeful and inspiring. Other times, you may find it depressing. As you will see, a vast array of emotional experiences and reactions are to be expected following a reproductive loss. My hope is that you will find something from this book to help soften but also to help you accept each of these emotional experiences. It is my privilege to go along with you on your journey to healing, self-care, and personal growth.

CHAPTER 1

NORMALIZING EMOTIONAL EXPERIENCES

There is no doubt that the fallout from a reproductive loss is brutal. If you required medical treatment at a hospital, it is excruciating to leave without your baby. If you were far enough along to feel movement and your baby kicking, the emptiness in your womb that follows can seem unbearable. If you had been trying to get pregnant for much longer than you had expected, the heartache can be gut-wrenching. Regardless of the specific circumstances surrounding your reproductive loss, you are experiencing the loss of an important dream that is central to your identity as a person who hopes to start or expand your family.

As devastating as it is, know that the first several weeks following the loss or trauma are the absolute worst. It does get better, slowly, over time. You will not stay in this limbo forever, even though, at the moment, it feels like you will. In this chapter, I describe the myriad emotions that you might be experiencing during this difficult period of your life, as well as some thoughts that go with those emotions and ways you might be handling those emotions and thoughts. The point of outlining these for you is to communicate that what you are experiencing is to be expected, however intense or out of character it feels.

EMOTIONAL EXPERIENCES IN THE FIRST WEEKS

There are no right or wrong emotions to feel during this time; everyone is different. In fact, it is quite possible that you will find yourself experiencing a variety of emotions at once or moving quickly from one intense emotional state to a completely different, but equally intense, one. During the first weeks following a reproductive loss, it might seem like your emotions are on a roller-coaster and that you can't imagine you will ever feel "normal" again.

These emotional experiences are compounded by physiological changes you may be experiencing. If you were taking fertility medications, many of your hormone levels are "out-of-whack." If you experienced a first trimester miscarriage, not only will your hormone levels be shifting back to baseline, but you also might be experiencing bleeding, cramping, and possible infection. If you had an incomplete miscarriage, you might be waiting to see whether you need surgical intervention. The further along you were in your pregnancy, the more likely it is that you are producing breast milk—a cruel reminder of the loss that you have experienced. Other physical symptoms you may be experiencing include anemia, night sweats, and hearing your pulse in your ear. Although the precise manner in which these physiological changes affect emotional experiences is unclear, the end result is that you are not feeling well physically, which can further sap the psychological resources that you would normally use to cope with adversity.

In the following sections, I describe some of the emotions that you may be experiencing in the first weeks following your reproductive loss.

Numbness

Many people who have experienced a reproductive loss report feeling numb at first, as if they can't feel anything. If you had a procedure in a hospital, it might have seemed like a whirlwind, leaving little time to acknowledge or experience emotions, let alone make sense of them. Those feelings of numbness and unreality can persist for several days after you have returned home. It might seem as if the possibility of ever experiencing joy and happiness again is nonexistent. Trust me, it just seems that way—you will feel joy and happiness again, although it might not be for some time. Also, some of the joy and happiness might take on new meaning.

Disbelief

Other people who have experienced a reproductive loss report a sense of disbelief. "Did that just happen?" It might seem like one moment you were pregnant and planning for a new addition to the family, and the next minute you were left with nothing. It also can be difficult to comprehend an entirely new view of one's reproductive health. For example, many women who have experienced a pregnancy loss will be considered at risk in future pregnancies and will receive additional monitoring and intervention. They may have never entertained the notion that they would be regarded as at risk in pregnancy. In the first weeks following a pregnancy loss, it is often difficult to accept that childbearing might always be different, and more difficult, for you than it is for women at low risk. Your new reality might be quite different from the reproductive story that you had envisioned for yourself.

Profound Sadness

There are usually a lot of tears in the first weeks following a reproductive loss. Many people describe a profound sadness unlike anything they have ever experienced before. This sadness might even be accompanied by a sense of hopelessness about the future, lack of interest in your routine and activities that you used to enjoy, sleep disturbance (either sleeping fitfully or sleeping too much), appetite disturbance (either having little appetite or overeating), fatigue, and difficulty concentrating. Reproductive loss can really hit a person's self-esteem, even to the point at which she might experience a sense of worthlessness. Some women recall a profound sense of inadequacy following a reproductive loss—after all, "if I can't even do something that it seems like all other women can do—have a child—what good am I?" Men can have the same reaction, especially if they are struggling with male infertility. Other people report pervasive, excessive guilt over the fact that they could not do anything to save the unborn child. Still others believe that the reproductive loss is a punishment for past transgressions. At times, it might seem like life is not worth living.

All of the experiences that I described in the previous paragraph are those that can contribute to a diagnosis of depression—major depression, to be exact. However, I want to be clear that grieving a substantial loss, such as a pregnancy loss, is absolutely normal and in no way means that you have a disorder. It also does not mean that you absolutely must receive professional mental health services. In fact, much of the material that I include in this book will help you to process the loss and heal on your own. In the final section of this chapter, I provide some guidelines for determining when consultation with a mental health professional is warranted.

Guilt

Although I mentioned guilt previously in the section on sadness, it is worth noting that guilt can take on a life of its own following a reproductive loss. As stated previously, many women feel significant guilt that they were unable to save or otherwise take care of their baby. If you were under anesthesia when the fetus was removed, you might feel guilt that you were not present for the moments when your baby was alive. Women often feel guilt associated with their belief that they have failed to give their partner a child; men often feel guilt associated with their belief that they should do more to help their partner and their child. People who have experienced reproductive loss and trauma often fixate on the idea that the loss is somehow their fault or that they should have done more to prevent it. The tools described in this book will help you put this guilt in perspective.

Anger and Envy

If the profound sadness and guilt aren't enough, many people who have experienced a reproductive loss speak of the pronounced anger that they endure, which often translates into envy of others who seem to so easily have gotten the perfect child or family. Despite what the statistics say, after enduring a pregnancy loss or reproductive trauma, it feels as if you are the only one who has had to go through something like this and that everyone else has had it so much easier. "It's not fair" pops up over and over in your mind, even if you are a person who otherwise takes the good with the bad and has the capacity to understand that bad things happen to good people, often for no apparent reason. It doesn't help that the media bombard us with the excruciating details of the blissful pregnancies and childbirths of public figures who were hard partying and irresponsible when they conceived. "What did I do to deserve this? How come they deserve to have a child, and I don't?"

It's worth noting that many people who have experienced reproductive loss describe another round of guilt associated with their anger and envy. "I'm not a person like this. I've never wanted anything but the best for other people." The anger and envy might catch you off guard because these feelings are so inconsistent with the person you believe yourself to be. You might feel guilty because you believe you are being mean-spirited toward others, and you might wonder whether you are turning into an angry, bitter person. Know that many, many people who have experienced reproductive loss have the same emotional experiences, and know that they soften over time. They do not define you and they will not define who you are in the long term.

Anger can manifest in different forms as well. People who have experienced reproductive loss might feel anger toward their spouses, bosses, or others whom they perceived pushed them too hard. They might feel anger toward medical staff whom they perceived as not taking their concerns seriously enough. Some obstetricians don't even schedule appointments with women until they are at least 12 weeks along in their pregnancies, leaving people who experience first trimester losses to feel invalidated and unacknowledged. There is also a general sense of anger toward a system that can't do more to intervene. For example, people who experience neonatal losses between 20 and 24.5 weeks are usually told by obstetricians and neonatologists that their babies are not viable and that it would be better if these babies did not live. Such comments can be experienced as insensitive and cold to expectant parents who have watched the fetus grow over the past several months and who so desperately want a family.

Loneliness

Many women who experience first-trimester losses have not yet announced their pregnancies to others. They often report an internal struggle over whether to share the news of the loss. A profound sense of loneliness can result when these people are in a position in which virtually nobody knows of their authentic experience in the moment. Loneliness is also experienced by people who have losses at any stage during pregnancy or who are going through unsuccessful fertility treatments, as they often look around at others who have the family composition for which they are longing. It can feel almost as if they are living outside of accepted social norms.

Apprehension About the Future

Not surprisingly, people who experience a reproductive loss have a great deal of apprehension about the future. "Was there permanent damage done to my reproductive organs? Will I ever conceive again, and if I do, will I be able to carry to full term? Will I ever have a family?" Although the practice of medicine has its basis in science, much of conception and pregnancy, especially during the first trimester of pregnancy, takes a wait-and-see approach. Women who undergo fertility treatments, such as in vitro fertilization, are closely monitored during conception and the first trimester of pregnancy, and even then, physicians really can't do much of anything if the pregnancy is not going to work out.

The heart of the apprehension is the uncertainty of all of it. The future—the ability to conceive, the ability to carry full-term, the ultimate number of children one might have—is uncertain. All of us, and especially people who have experienced reproductive loss, must find ways to accept, deal with, and even embrace uncertainty in our lives. There are no guarantees. And that can be the hardest thing to face in the weeks following a reproductive loss.

EMOTIONAL EXPERIENCES AFTER THE FIRST WEEKS

Eventually, you will resume many of your usual activities—you'll go back to work, maintain your household, pay your bills, and so on. This does not mean, however, that you are expected to be completely "back to normal." As I state on many occasions in this book, a reproductive loss is an experience that remains with many people in some form or another throughout their lives. I'm not saying this to be fatalistic—you will figure out how to live a quality, meaningful, and satisfying life in light of this devastating experience. I say this to reassure you that you are not expected to simply "get over" or forget about the loss. You will likely create a "new normal" (see Chapters 3 and 10), such that you integrate the loss into your outlook on life in a healthy, adaptive, and balanced manner.

However, the new normal takes time to establish. Thus, in this section, I describe some of the emotional experiences described by people after the first postloss weeks have passed but before they have achieved that new normal.

Bouts of Acute Emotional Distress

You might find that, over time, your emotional distress (i.e., depression, anxiety, anger) might lessen. Then, suddenly, you are overcome by one or more of these emotions and are experiencing them just as acutely as you did during the first few weeks following the loss or trauma. Sometimes these emotions have logical triggers—you see a baby while you are out shopping, you stumble upon a baby gift that someone had given you, or you learn that yet another friend is pregnant. But, at times, these bouts seem to come out of the blue, leaving you to wonder whether something is really wrong with you. Sometimes others will not understand why you are so upset; after all, in their view, you had been doing pretty well for several weeks now.

These intense bouts of emotion are understandable, even if they occur many weeks, months, and even years after the reproductive loss. In many cases, these bouts are part of the ups and downs of the grieving process. They can be discouraging; many people who have experienced reproductive loss indicate that they just want their lives to go back to the way they used to be and wonder when this will be over. As long as these bouts are not causing substantial life interference or are associated with intent to harm yourself, I encourage you not to attach excessive significance to them—they do not necessarily mean that you are going crazy or that something is terribly wrong with you. Accepting your emotional experience in the moment, whatever it is, letting go of the struggle against it, and refraining from reading too much into it can enhance your overall psychological well-being. In other words, you can just let your emotions and thoughts be. I say more about ways to do this in Chapter 9.

Avoidance of Painful Reminders

There is no doubt that being in the presence of pregnant women and young children reopens the still-fresh wound of the reproductive loss. It can bring on the acute bouts of emotional distress described in the previous section. It can also bring on more chronic feelings of despair and emptiness. These chronic feelings are often accompanied by thoughts such as "I'll never have a baby," "This is never going to happen for me," and even "I'm less of a woman (or man) than other people." Not surprisingly, these emotions and thoughts can be associated with urges to avoid pregnant women and young children. Doing so, however, can be especially difficult when you have a family member or close friend who is pregnant or who has young children, or if you have coworkers who are pregnant or who have young children and it is part of your job to interact with them on a regular basis. Painful reminders of the reproductive loss are also triggered by gynecological visits, sometimes even years after the loss. Some women report enduring these visits with extreme dread or avoiding them altogether because they are afraid that painful wounds would be reopened.

It is not abnormal to want to avoid these painful reminders. On the contrary, it makes a lot of sense—it's human nature to make great efforts to avoid pain and despair. Over time, you will figure out the best way for you to cope with these reminders. I present a framework for overcoming avoidance of these reminders in Chapter 7.

Fixation on the Loss

Many people who have experienced reproductive loss continue to pay keen attention to time in relation to their pregnancy. You might note that, at this point, you would have been, say, 28 weeks along in your pregnancy, 30 weeks along in your pregnancy, and so on. You might visit pregnancy websites and contemplate the symptoms you'd be experiencing at this point in the pregnancy. Understandably, the baby's due date is an especially difficult day and is one in which you can expect to experience an exacerbation of emotional distress. However, even after the baby's due date, you may find yourself noting how old the baby would be at that point in time and think about the manner in which the baby would be developing, what the baby would be doing at that age, and what the baby would look like. All of this occurs with a sense of wistfulness and remorse. To complicate matters further, others may not understand this urge to track what the baby's development would have been, which can leave you with the sense that you are alone and misunderstood.

Remembering and acknowledging your child can be an important part of the grieving process. However, it is crucial to ensure that this remembering and acknowledging is working *for* you, rather than *against* you. If you find that this remembering and acknowledging takes up a substantial portion of time and gets in the way of other life activities, it might have developed into rumination that is prolonging your suffering, rather than helping you work through it. In Chapter 10, I describe ways to commemorate your child that others have found to facilitate their grief in a healthy manner.

More Apprehension

After one or more months following the reproductive loss have passed, you might have medical clearance to begin trying again. But trying again brings more anxiety and apprehension. I have never met a pregnant woman who didn't have at least a little bit of anxiety, and that anxiety increases exponentially when she has experienced a previous loss or trauma. "What if's" are common as you are trying again—most of them boil down to "what if I experience another loss?" There are no guarantees as to if and when you will get pregnant again. And if you do get pregnant, 40 or more weeks of pregnancy can seem excruciating.

If you decide not to try to get pregnant again, you might experience continued apprehension in a different way. Although the end result is gratifying, the adoption process can be stressful and uncertain. "What if we opt for adoption, and the birth mother suddenly decides that she does not want to go through with it? What if we adopt a baby who is genetically predisposed to a certain illness?" If you choose not to have children, you might wonder whether you will have regrets at a later time. "What if we don't have children and then have no one to take care of us when we are older?"

Regardless of whether you try to get pregnant again (on your own or with the help of fertility treatments), initiate the adoption process, or decide to live your life without children, you will be faced with apprehension and what if's." You will not get rid of the what if's. But you can learn to get distance from them, gain perspective on them, accept that they are simply thoughts that can be let be, and live a valued life in spite of your anxiety and apprehension. The tools described in many of the subsequent chapters will help you to do that.

Limbo

Along with the apprehension about your reproductive future is a sense of limbo. Many people who have experienced reproductive loss are just ready to be done with childbearing and to know what their family composition will be. Instead, they are faced with what could be years of uncertainty. It might feel as if the appointments, planning, dreaming, and even longing are never ending. You might find that your major decisions need to be put on hold, such as whether to buy a larger house, whether to move closer to extended family, whether to change to a different health insurance benefit, or whether to take a job that is demanding or one that is flexible. Some people find that they are paralyzed by even small decisions (e.g., "Should I work hard to lose weight? It will all be for naught if I just get pregnant again"). It can feel maddening. It is important to go into this period of your life with eyes wide open, knowing that you will be in this state of limbo for a while.

Vacillation

In the many weeks and months after a reproductive loss, you might find yourself struggling to achieve acceptance—of the loss, of the uncertainty, and of the possibility that your reproductive story might not play out as you had hoped. As you proceed on your journey toward acceptance, you may find yourself vacillating among a number of emotional experiences, as well as among decisions about the future that you may be contemplating. One day, you might feel good about life again, being able to "smell the roses" and appreciate the many aspects of your life that seem to be going well. The very next day, you might experience one of those bouts of emotional distress and focus on all that has gone wrong for you. One day, you might have the sense that it is OK that you might not have children or that you might not have as many children as you had hoped. The very next day, you might be consumed with childbearing and believe that the only thing that will ever make you feel whole is to have a child (or another child). The path to acceptance is not a linear one, and this vacillation is to be expected.

Childbearing carries profound meaning for women and men, alike. No one expects you to make a firm decision while you are healing from a reproductive loss. For that matter, even people who have not experienced such losses often vacillate on their thoughts and feelings about how, if, and when to have children. You are allowed to feel differently at different times. You might even feel paralyzed by the vacillation, unable to move in one direction or another. This sense of paralysis will loosen over time as you become more comfortable with the direction in which you move with your acceptance.

Dread

Underlying many of the emotional experiences discussed thus far is a vague sense of dread. "What if I can't have the life that I had envisioned for myself?" There is perhaps no greater threat to one's sense of meaning and purpose than facing possibility that one cannot have in life the things that are most precious and cherished. A reproductive loss or trauma does not have to mean that you will never have a child. That being said, your circumstances might be such that you need to redefine or reshape your view of a meaningful and purposeful life. Chapters 3 and 10 say more about this. A basic premise of this book is that you can live a fulfilling, meaningful life consistent with your values and strengths, no matter how your reproductive story plays out.

ACUTE AND COMPLICATED GRIEF

Over the past decade, there has been increasing attention devoted to the scientific study of grief. According to renowned scholar M. Katherine Shear and her colleagues, *acute grief* is commonly experienced following the loss of a loved one, and it is characterized by a sense of disbelief, difficulty accepting the death, painful emotions, prominent and preoccupying memories of the deceased, and lack of engagement in life's activities. Shear's research found that, in most cases, after six months, the bereaved move into a period of *integrated grief*, characterized by acceptance of the death, memories of the deceased that arise from time to time but that are not preoccupying, a reestablishment of interest and engagement in life, and the predominant experience of positive emotions. *Complicated grief*, in contrast, is characterized by prolonged and indefinite acute grief accompanied by intrusive thoughts and images of the death, rumination over the death, and avoidance of reminders of the death. Shear's research has demonstrated that complicated grief can be treated successfully with psychotherapy.

The degree to which this model applies to people who have experienced reproductive loss, however, is unclear. Although at least one research study has examined the course of complicated grief associated with the death of a child (average age a little older than 5), no available research has examined complicated grief in people who have experienced miscarriage or neonatal loss. Moreover, a key feature of healthy grief seems to be the adaptive coping with memories of the deceased. In fact, Ruth Malkinson, author of a book describing a cognitive behavioral approach to bereavement, summarizes research suggesting that healthy grievers eventually form adaptive and continued bonds with the deceased. This aspect of bereavement is not relevant to people who have experienced pregnancy loss, as they have few, if any memories of their child. They didn't know their child. Here again is another instance in which the grief process of people who have experienced reproductive loss is different from that of people who have experienced other types of losses. Whether or not this difference prolongs the grief in people who have experienced reproductive loss hasn't yet been determined.

WHAT IF MY EMOTIONAL EXPERIENCES SEEM WRONG?

Many people who have experienced reproductive loss are surprised by the intensity of their emotional experiences and become concerned when they view these emotional experiences as out of character for them. It also doesn't help when others make comments to the tune that you "should" be feeling, thinking, or doing something differently. I've encountered family members of people who have experienced reproductive loss who had great empathy for the pain that the individual experienced immediately following the loss but who later began to wonder when their loved one would "move on." When family members and close others harbor these opinions, it is likely that they will be communicated in subtle ways. This just contributes to the person's sense of isolation and distance from others.

Keep these important points in mind when you begin to wonder whether there is something wrong with you:

- There is no "right" way to grieve a reproductive loss.
- It is absolutely understandable that you feel the way you do.
- There are constant triggers that reopen the wound again and again and again and again.
- You will begin to get perspective and make meaning from the situation when you are able to do so.

Read these statements over and over.

WHEN IS PROFESSIONAL HELP WARRANTED?

Despite reading the material in this chapter, you might still be concerned that something is wrong with you. The following are some warning signs that suggest professional help may be beneficial and even warranted:

- Have you been staying in bed all day, every day, for several weeks? As I discuss in Chapter 2 of this volume, some degree of inactivity, isolation, and "holing up" is normal following a reproductive loss. However, eventually these coping strategies will be counterproductive because they will prevent you from having the kinds of experiences that will facilitate the grieving process. If you feel like you cannot get out of bed or reengage after several weeks have passed, it may be time to think about seeking professional help.

- Are your emotional experiences interfering with your ability to work, take care of your other children, or engage in basic self-care for yourself? No one would expect you to be functioning at 100% for many, many weeks after a reproductive loss. However, if, after several weeks have passed, your emotional experiences are causing substantial life interference that prevents you from completing life's basic and necessary tasks, it may be time to think about seeking professional help.

- Are you having frequent and intrusive flashbacks of or nightmares about the loss? Research shows that a substantial proportion of women view relatively straightforward labor and delivery as traumatic, such that they feared that they or their baby would be harmed or would die. It makes sense, then, that an acute loss event in which your baby indeed did not live would be experienced as traumatic. If these intrusive flashbacks and nightmares are interfering with your ability to function or with your emotional well-being, you might consider seeking help from a professional who specializes in the treatment of posttraumatic stress. In Chapter 4, I briefly describe the way cognitive behavioral treatment for these symptoms works.

- Do you have any intent to act on suicidal thoughts, or do you have a plan in place to harm yourself? As stated previously, it is common for people who have had a reproductive loss to have thoughts like life isn't worth living and that they would be better off dead. You might even have thoughts like, "I wish

I were dead." Suicidal thoughts become particularly concerning when people have intent to act on the suicidal thoughts or have developed a specific plan for hurting themselves. If you or your partner have persistent suicidal thoughts, suicidal intent, or a suicide plan, it is important to contact a mental health professional immediately.

- Are you engaging in any other self-destructive acts? Examples of these acts could include harming yourself without the intent of killing yourself (e.g., cutting yourself), excessive alcohol or drug use that puts you or others at risk of harm, bingeing and purging, promiscuity, and spending money beyond your means. In these cases, professional help could help you to develop more adaptive coping skills that do not put you or your family at risk.

As I stated in the Introduction, choosing a mental health professional can be tricky because many have not received specific training in perinatal issues. It might be tempting instead to contact your obstetrician, with the idea that this individual would have a better understanding of your recent loss. For some people, this is a great option because obstetricians have dealt with many, many people who have experienced reproductive losses and have been privy to the pain that it causes. However, many obstetricians are not trained in mental health, and unfortunately, some address only the most cursory emotional and psychological needs. One of my clients remembers being extremely tearful during her 6-week post-loss appointment with an obstetrician after she had been waiting in the waiting room for over an hour with a room full of pregnant (and seemingly healthy) women. The obstetrician saw the tears and immediately said quite bluntly, "You need to go to therapy" rather than empathizing with the experience she had just had in the waiting room. Not surprisingly, she left the appointment feeling miserable, perceiving that she had been judged and dismissed, and wondering whether her emotional reaction was inappropriate and silly. Thus, the obstetrician is a logical place to start seeking assistance; however, if you receive a response that does not seem particularly compassionate, know that this has happened in the past and that there are other places to turn.

How does one go about finding a mental health professional who has training, experience, and sensitivity in working with perinatal issues? Fortunately, there are specific societies, resources, and treatment centers that are devoted to perinatal issues, thanks to the massive attention that postpartum depression has received over the past two decades. Although grief associated with a reproductive loss is not the same as postpartum depression, mental health providers who specialize in postpartum depression will almost assuredly be a good match for these issues because of their knowledge of perinatal issues in general. A first step in finding a clinician who specializes in postpartum depression, or more generally in perinatal psychology, would be to contact the Internet site of Postpartum Support International (http://www.postpartum.net). By clicking on the "get help" menu, you will see a map of the United States where you can click on your state and get the name of a regional coordinator who will be familiar with resources in your area. You can also visit one of many therapist directories (e.g., http://www.psychologytoday.com and http://locator.apa.org) and read through the profiles of therapists in your area. Therapists who specialize in treating perinatal women will often indicate so on these profiles. Keep in mind, however, that the information that can be included on these profiles is usually not regulated, so you will want to verify that the clinician indeed has expertise in perinatal psychology.

Even if the warning signs I listed previously do not characterize your experience, it is OK to seek professional help if you believe that it would be helpful to you. Perhaps you have been in therapy in the past and found it helpful, and you'd like to reconnect with that therapist. Perhaps you perceive that others in your support network do not understand what you are going through, and you think a professional would be able to meet that need. Perhaps you'd like face-to-face contact with someone to walk you through tools similar to those described in this book. The main message is that you are allowed to take the path to healing that is right for you and that you might stroll down many paths before you find the right fit.

Some people worry that if they seek help from a mental health professional, they will be hospitalized in a psychiatric ward against their will. In actuality, this occurrence is very, very rare. Hospitalization is warranted when a person indicates that she is at imminent risk of harming herself or others, with *imminent* usually defined as harm occurring in the next 24 to 48 hours. Unless you are at imminent risk, simply telling a mental health provider that you have suicidal thoughts will not necessarily land you in a hospital. These thoughts are part of the grieving process, and there are many courses of action that you and your mental health provider can decide on in a collaborative manner, such as having more than one therapy session per week or informing your spouse that you are having these thoughts so that your spouse can monitor you for safety.

I have also encountered people who have experienced reproductive loss who are not suicidal but who are consumed with sadness and anxiety, leaving them to wonder whether they are going crazy and need to be hospitalized. Some women who have other children at home worry that these children will be taken away from them because they are going crazy. Experiencing intense emotions, even emotions that seem out of control, will not land you in a hospital unless you are engaging in risky behavior that puts you or others in harm's way. Interestingly, the fact that you are worrying about going crazy is actually a good sign because it indicates that you recognize that your emotions and thoughts are unwanted and inconsistent with who you are—it is more concerning when a person is behaving bizarrely but is unaware that her behavior is out of character or is convinced that the behavior is appropriate. The message I give my clients is, "You're not going crazy. You're reacting to a tragic, tragic experience that I wish you didn't have to go through."

IN A NUTSHELL

After a reproductive loss, you might experience emotions unlike those you've ever experienced in your life. They can be intense, they can be scary, and they can make you wonder whether you're going crazy. Although you will gradually resume your usual activities and get back to your routine, you will continue to have the sense that things have changed. The world that seemed generally safe, predictable, and fair will seem much less so. The "rules" of bereavement may not seem to apply to you.

At this point, you may be wondering how you will ever feel whole again, feel happiness again, or feel hope for the future. I'm reminded here of a quotation by Helen Keller: "Character cannot be developed in ease and quiet. Only through experience of trial and suffering can the soul be strengthened, ambition inspired, and success achieved." Inspired by this quotation, I sometimes ask my clients, "If you have to be in this awful situation, how can you endure it with grace and dignity, achieving personal growth along the way?" Many of my clients have told me that the "grace and dignity" phrase runs over and over in their minds as they cope with their loss.

Even if this rings true for you, believe me, there will be times when you feel anything but graceful and dignified. I certainly lacked grace and dignity at many, many points along my healing journey. But this phrase can serve as a guiding principle that will ultimately help you to find meaning from your tragic experience. And it may help you to embrace some of the tools that I describe in the subsequent chapters of this volume, which when they are implemented, will make it that much easier to weather this experience with grace and dignity. Many years from now, when you look back on this experience, you will be surprised at the inner strength that you cultivated during your healing. Renowned psychologist George Bonanno has found the most common outcome following a loss or potentially traumatic event is that of resilience. I offer you the tools described in this book to forge your own path toward resilience.

CHAPTER 2

GETTING BY IN THE FIRST WEEKS

It's all well and good to understand that your emotional experiences are to be expected, but most people who have experienced reproductive loss want to know what to do about the enormous distress that they are enduring. In this chapter, I present some things you can do right now to take care of yourself and set yourself up to begin the healing process. Many of these strategies are not long-term strategies that will resolve the grief and emotional experiences on their own. However, they will be especially useful in getting you through difficult moments, which will help build resilience every time you use them and center you so that you can ultimately face the grief and decisions you might need to make. They also provide the foundation for the use of the other strategies described in this book.

SELF-CARE: A MUST

You probably will not feel like doing much to take care of yourself in the weeks after a reproductive loss. And during those few weeks, you can give yourself permission not to engage in perfect self-care. You just need to do what you can to get by.

After that, though, you still won't be feeling anywhere close to your usual self, but it will be essential to begin taking care of yourself. That's the case whether or not you have resumed your other usual activities—work, school, volunteer work, and so on. In other words, it is understandable that you probably won't be functioning anywhere close to 100% after the first few weeks following a reproductive loss, but it nevertheless is time for you to start taking small steps toward self-care. In this section, I describe several aspects of self-care to which it is important to attend. Although they may seem basic and self-evident, when I ask my clients how well they are attending to these aspects of self-care, I find that they usually are neglecting several, if not all of the areas, which has the potential to disrupt the grieving process.

I view self-care as a pie chart, with each piece of the pie representing a behavior that contributes to the overall pie of optimal self-care (see Figure 2.1). Think of it this way: Even if one or two of the pieces of your pie chart are not yet in order, the other pieces of the pie can carry you through until you can attend to them. However, if all of the pieces of your pie are not yet in order, then it is possible that this first period of emotionally intense grieving and despair will be prolonged. No one is perfect, but even having a few of the pieces of your self-care pie in place will ultimately help you to develop the inner resources to continue on your healing journey.

Sleep

It is easy for one's sleep cycle to become disrupted, such that one sleeps a great deal during the day and is awake all night. We know that there is a two-way association between sleep and aversive emotional experiences, like sadness and anxiety. This means that sleep disturbance can certainly be caused and exacerbated by sadness and anxiety but that sleep disturbance, in and of itself, can make sadness

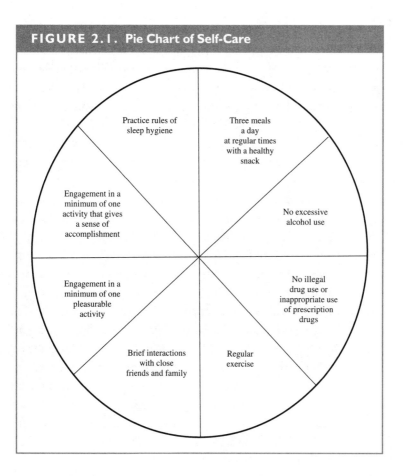

FIGURE 2.1. Pie Chart of Self-Care

Practice rules of
sleep hygiene

Three meals
a day
at regular times
with a healthy
snack

Engagement in a
minimum of one
activity that gives
a sense of
accomplishment

No excessive
alcohol use

Engagement in a
minimum of one
pleasurable
activity

No illegal
drug use or
inappropriate use
of prescription
drugs

Brief interactions
with close
friends and family

Regular
exercise

and anxiety worse. As much as you feel like sleeping during the day, and as much as you are drained by sleepless nights, it is critical for you to attend to your sleep and take action to ensure that you are getting the rest and the restoration that you need. Unfortunately, there is no specific number of hours of sleep that you should target; everyone is different. You know yourself better than anyone—what is the optimal number of hours of sleep you'd be getting each night to feel rested and centered the next day? It may be 7 hours a night; it may be 9 hours a night. Whatever is right for you, that's what you should target, as long as it is within reason. Sleep expert Michael Perlis suggested that anything less than 6 or 6.5 hours per night is problematic.

Exhibit 2.1 lists some rules of sleep hygiene. *Sleep hygiene* is a lot like dental hygiene—just as it is important to have regular visits with your dentists, brush your teeth twice a day, and floss, it is equally as important to engage in regular habits that promote healthy sleep. By following these rules and incorporating them into your daily routine, you will likely find that not only will you sleep better, you will also be more centered, rested, and able to take on the challenges of the next day. What's more, staying up late at night, perhaps when your partner has already gone to bed, creates a situation that is ripe for unhelpful rumination about the loss or trauma. One of my clients referred to this time as the "witching hour," such that when she was alone late at night thinking about her loss, she was invariably overcome with intrusive thoughts, self-doubt, and despair. More often than not, when she finally went to bed, she was in tears and woke her partner in the middle of the night to be comforted.

Sleep hygiene works in a number of ways. First, it gives you the best shot possible to have a good night's sleep. By ensuring that your bedroom is dark, quiet, and at a comfortable temperature, you are increasing the likelihood that extraneous factors will not wake you during the night. By refraining from eating a heavy meal, drinking alcohol, smoking, and exercising in the hours leading up to bedtime, you increase the likelihood that your body will be in a resting state that will facilitate the onset of sleep. By only using your bed for sleep and sex, maintaining a regular bedtime routine, maintaining a regular sleep schedule, and getting out of bed when you are lying awake for more than a half hour, you will condition your body to expect sleep at a certain time and maximize the amount of cues that will signal your body that it is time to go to sleep. In other words, when you

EXHIBIT 2.1. Rules of Sleep Hygiene

- Set a regular sleep schedule (i.e., regular time to bed, regular time to wake) and stick with it 7 days a week.
- Avoid naps.
- Use the bed only for sleep and sex. Do not read, watch television, talk on the phone, or eat in bed.
- Go to bed only when you are very sleepy.
- Engage in a relaxing activity an hour before bedtime. No working or answering e-mails.
- Develop a predictable bedtime routine (e.g., washing face, brushing teeth) to serve as a cue that it is bedtime.
- If you are awake for longer than a half hour, get out of bed and engage in a quiet, nonarousing activity (no computer, phone, or tablet device) until you feel sleepy enough to go back to bed.
- Turn the clock so that you cannot see it.
- Do not turn on smartphones or tablet devices in the middle of the night. Consider storing smartphones or tablet devices outside of the bedroom if their flickering lights keep you awake.
- Refrain from drinking caffeinated beverages after noon.
- Refrain from using alcohol as a sleep aid.
- If you smoke, decrease the amount of cigarettes you smoke in the evening and refrain from smoking in the evening altogether if you can.
- Exercise regularly but do not do so within 4 hours of bedtime.
- Do not fixate on sleeping a certain number of hours.
- Make sure your bedroom is dark, quiet, and at a comfortable temperature. Use a white noise machine to minimize noise if you need to do so.
- Make sure your bed is comfortable.
- Do not go to bed hungry but do not eat a heavy meal before bed. A light snack before bed is fine.
- Avoid excessive intake of all liquids in the evening to avoid multiple bathroom trips in the middle of the night.
- Use the strategies described in this book to minimize the degree to which you are taking your problems, sadness, or anxiety to bed.

Note. Many of these sleep hygiene rules can be found in Hauri and Linde (1996); Perlis, Jungquist, Smith, and Posner (2005); and Silberman (2008).

implement the principles of sleep hygiene, you are paving the way for the establishment of healthy habits that will last a lifetime. Moreover, it will give you a sense of control over one aspect of your life when other areas of your life feel like they are out of control.

There may be times when you feel frustrated because you *are* following the principles of sleep hygiene, and you're still having trouble sleeping. It's likely that the sadness and anxiety are continuing to interfere with your sleep. This can be especially true in people who have a history of sleep disturbance. My suggestion to you is to keep trying—don't give up on the principles of sleep hygiene because they are unquestionably the foundation of healthy sleep. As silly as this might sound, know that your body will not let you go without sleep forever. The longer you are awake, the more you build up *sleep debt*, which means that your body feels increasingly fatigued and experiences more and more pressure for sleep. You might have to temper your expectations that you'll sleep for as many hours or as soundly as you'd like to sleep. But know that you *will* sleep. Many of my clients also find it comforting to know that research shows that people who struggle with sleep disturbance sleep more than they think they do. They perceive that they are awake for significant periods of time, but in reality, they are in and out of sleep and are indeed getting some rest.

When you have trouble sleeping, you may start to panic. You may look at the clock and do mental arithmetic to calculate the maximum number of hours of sleep you will get from that point forward. You may start to think about all of the ways you will be affected the next day if you do not get enough sleep and are tired. You may focus on how badly you are going to feel the next day if you are unable to sleep. Interestingly, sleep experts indicate that it is especially common for people to experience such panic-ridden thoughts in the middle of the night because the prefrontal cortex of our brains (i.e., the part of the brain that is responsible for logical and goal-directed thought) is one of the first areas of the brain to fall asleep at night. This means that even if you feel as if you are awake, your prefrontal cortex is not functioning optimally, which provides a context that is ripe for the emergence of exaggerated and unrealistic thoughts. Many of my clients have told me that they answer these thoughts by saying to themselves, "These thoughts are just a result of my prefrontal cortex slowing down. They are not based in logic or fact."

If you are a person who tends to panic in the middle of the night when you have trouble sleeping, it could help to develop a *decatastrophizing statement* to put your mind at ease and remind yourself that the consequences of lack of sleep are not as catastrophic as your mind believes in the moment. Such a statement can provide the logic and facts that your mind might be forgetting when the frontal cortex is slowing down. The decatastrophizing statement was especially helpful for Angela, who had a history of insomnia and was experiencing an especially troubling bout of sleep disturbance after her reproductive loss. Her decatastrophizing statement read as follows: "I know I will get at least SOME sleep tonight because I always fall asleep eventually. And I know that research shows that many people sleep more than they think they do. I've had plenty of times in my life when I've only gotten a few hours of sleep, and while I'm tired the next day, I've always been able to do what I need to do. So, not getting a lot of sleep tonight is unfortunate, but it's not a catastrophe."

One issue to consider with decatastrophizing statements is how you will consult it in the middle of the night when the room is dark. Turning on the light might make you more awake, and if you aren't sleeping alone, might disturb your partner. Many people identify the creative solution of storing the decatastrophizing statement on their smartphone or tablet device. Although this solution allows for easy access to the statement, the problem is that turning on the device allows the backlight to shine right into your face, which has the potential to be activating and make you more awake. To avoid these problems, I suggest that you develop your decatastrophizing statement during the daytime, when it is light and you can put some thought into it. Then, I recommend that you read it right before you turn the lights off and go to bed. Read the statement every night so that you are familiar with it; in that way, you eliminate the need to turn on a source of light to read the statement. However, there very well might be times when the decatastrophizing statement will have the greatest effect when you read it directly. One rule of sleep hygiene is to get out of bed and engage in a quiet activity if you have been lying awake for more than a half hour. Perhaps you can keep your decatastrophizing statement in the location in which you engage in your quiet activity.

Although difficulty sleeping can be a big problem for people who have experienced a reproductive loss, others experience the opposite problem—sleeping many, many more hours during the day than they would otherwise. Sleeping too much can be just as disruptive to your sleep cycle as not sleeping enough. If this describes you, it is likely that you set the alarm for 8, 9, or 10 hours later, the alarm rings, and you turn it off, feeling as if you weigh a million pounds and that nothing in the world is powerful enough to drag you out of bed. You probably feel like your body is not rested and that you need more sleep. You might even have thoughts like, "What's the point of getting up? I have nothing to look forward to today." Although these thoughts are understandable in the weeks following a reproductive loss, it is important to find a way to overcome them so that you are not sleeping excessively. Later in this chapter, I describe the importance of engaging in activities that are associated with a sense of pleasure and accomplishment and the importance of utilizing your social support network. Perhaps you can schedule one of these activities or a visit with someone in your social support network for an hour or two after you would get out of bed so that you have something to look forward to, or at least something that you will view as an appointment to which you will feel accountable. When the time comes, you won't necessarily feel like getting out of bed for these reasons, but they will serve the purpose of ensuring that you are sleeping a reasonable number of hours that won't throw off your sleep cycle.

Meals

Just like regular sleep, we need regular meals to maintain a healthy and stable physiological homeostasis, or equilibrium. It is possible that you will not feel like eating at all. However, it is just as possible that you will feel like eating all the time, and especially like eating foods that are not good for you. The rules of thumb are to eat three nutritious meals—breakfast, lunch, and dinner—and not to skip any of these meals, even if you are not that hungry. If you need a snack, by all means eat one, but be sure that it is nutritious (e.g., fruit, nuts, yogurt, crudités) and of a reasonable portion. One trick to make eating more appealing is to allow yourself to eat some of foods that you could not eat during pregnancy, such as brie cheese or deli meats.

Many people who have endured a loss or trauma have difficulty resuming a regular meal schedule because they simply don't know what they feel like eating. They open the refrigerator door, and nothing looks good. Or they are indecisive, having difficulty deciding whether they want to prepare something or whether they should just grab something easy. If this describes you, plan your meals in advance so that you don't need to deal with making a decision. Planning your meals might even be an enjoyable activity that you can do with your partner or a family member, as the two of you will likely be sharing some meals.

You might also be worried about your weight. One of the cruel realities of many miscarriages (i.e., loss through 20 weeks' gestation) and neonatal deaths (i.e., loss after 20 weeks' gestation) that occur when the fetus is still relatively tiny is that the baby weight does not come off as quickly as it does when one gives birth to a child. Moreover, weight gain is a side effect of some fertility drugs. In these first several weeks following a reproductive loss, give yourself permission not to worry about your weight. It's most important for you to get in the habit of eating healthy, nutritious meals. You can deal with dieting later, and when you are in a position to do so, you may actually find that it gives you a goal on which to focus your attention away from the reproductive loss. As you saw with sleep hygiene, eating regular and healthy meals is a habit that will serve as a foundation to maintaining a healthy weight in the future.

Alcohol

I will not say that I have a "no alcohol" rule following a reproductive loss, even though most responsible health professionals will recommend against using alcohol to cope or using alcohol when one is in a stage of her life in which she is trying to get pregnant. In fact, it can be a relatively innocuous simple pleasure to have a glass of wine after having abstained for an extended period of time. Thus, an occasional glass of wine or other alcoholic drink that you drink for the pleasure and enjoyment of doing so is OK; excessive alcohol use for the purpose of coping or escaping is not. Excessive alcohol use is associated with disturbed sleep, grogginess, and impaired concentration. These consequences are contrary to the self-care that I am encouraging in this chapter.

Drugs

Optimum self-care means no use of illegal drugs. It is possible that a physician or nurse practitioner has prescribed you a medicine for sleep (e.g., alprazolam) or for pain (e.g., oxycodone). As long as you are under the care the prescribing professional and using the medicines as they are intended, prescription medicines are fine to take and may actually help to ease the emotional and physical pain that you are experiencing. The idea is to use these drugs so that they enable you engage in healthy self-care, not to numb you or provide an escape that interferes with the implementation of self-care behaviors.

Exercise

Exercise is an important component of sleep hygiene. Regular exercise helps to regulate your physiological homeostasis, and a regular routine is important in ensuring that you get enough sleep each night. However, exercise has many benefits beyond its contribution to good sleep hygiene. When you exercise, chemicals called endorphins are released. Endorphins reduce the perception of pain, create an overall positive sensation in the body (think "runner's high"), and act as a sedative. In fact, psychologists Michael Otto and Jasper Smits found that exercise, in itself, can be a treatment for depression and anxiety or an important component in the multifaceted treatment of emotional distress. Thus, engaging in regular exercise has the potential to regulate your mood following a loss or trauma and even serve in a preventive capacity to reduce the likelihood of subsequent depression.

In addition, exercise has important health benefits and, perhaps more important, will give you the sense that you are doing something positive for yourself after having gone through an event that has the potential to wreak havoc on your body. Be sure to get clearance from your physician to implement exercise and be aware of any recommendations your physician might have for the degree to which you are able to exercise.

You might be thinking, "Yeah, right, easier said than done." You're tired. You're sad. Your body is not at its best. And you just don't feel like it. My suggestion is to start small and be creative to make exercise as enjoyable and as inviting as possible. Go for a walk at a scenic state park rather than pounding away on a treadmill at the gym. Go to a yoga or Pilates class at a soothing, inviting location outside the home, rather than using a DVD that you've already watched a million times. The point is that it is important to set yourself up for success, increasing the likelihood that you will follow through. Another important aspect of setting yourself up for success is to have reasonable expectations. Angela admitted that she avoided exercise because she used to win cross-country meets and was now disappointed that she could now barely run a mile without huffing and puffing. Give yourself permission to do only what your body tells you that it can do, and give yourself credit for engaging in any kind of exercise after the loss that you experienced.

Social Support

It is understandable that you will want to isolate yourself following a reproductive loss. It's hard to talk to extended family members who so very much were looking forward to a new addition to the family. It's hard to talk to friends who are pregnant or who have children. From a more general standpoint, it's hard to take that first step in making the first face-to-face or telephone contact with anyone who knows about the loss. You might be fearful that they will bring up the loss and that you will become emotional. You might be fearful that they will not bring up the loss and that you will be resentful. You might anticipate that the conversation will be awkward and just want to avoid it altogether.

In Chapter 6, I provide some hints for handling these specific conversations. Here, I will simply say that if, after the few weeks following a reproductive loss, you are still isolating yourself, please consider reaching out to the one or two people whom you anticipate will be the most helpful in providing support. Social support during times of loss, trauma, and grief is crucial in managing your distress and may even promote growth and healing. Moreover, like exercise, it has the potential to serve as a buffer against the development of problems such as depression and anxiety disorders.

So, think for a moment: Who makes you feel the most comfortable? Who has provided you helpful, nonjudgmental emotional support in the past? Who is invested in your emotional well-being but perhaps not so invested in the pregnancy that they are dealing with their own grief over the loss? These are the people who have the potential to be most helpful as you try to get by in the first weeks after a reproductive loss. You don't need to plan a major outing with these people. Simply talking on the phone or getting together for a quiet cup of tea at one of your homes will suffice.

Pleasurable Activities

According to behavioral theories of depression, such as that put forth more than 30 years ago by renowned psychologist Peter Lewinsohn, lack of engagement in activities that are enjoyable or that make you feel good creates a vicious cycle. On the one hand, when you are feeling down, it makes sense that you would want to lay low and hunker down so that you do not expend unnecessary energy—instead, you might sleep, mindlessly watch TV, or surf the Internet. However, when you forego engagement in activities that are truly pleasurable or enjoyable, you do not get much positive reinforcement from your environment. When that happens, it brings you down even further, thus lowering your energy and motivation to engage in pleasurable activities, which further decreases the likelihood that you will engage in these activities, which further decreases the likelihood that you will get positive reinforcement, and so on. By committing to engaging in one pleasurable activity per day, you will take a step in breaking free of this vicious cycle.

How do you know what activity to choose when nothing sounds good? It doesn't have to be an activity that involves a lot of planning, preparation, and coordination. The key is to experience a simple pleasure, not to take on a project that will end up overwhelming you. It could be something as simple as reading a fiction book that you've been wanting to read for a while or arranging a bouquet of flowers. In Chapter 3, I expand on these behavioral principles and show how they can help you to become more actively and meaningfully involved in your life in the later weeks following a reproductive loss. But for now, just choosing and implementing one simple but pleasurable activity will suffice. If you continue to have difficulty identifying something that you would find pleasurable, perhaps you can turn to the person in your social support network to whom you plan to reach out. Chances are, you have engaged in pleasurable activities in the past with that person, and he or she will be able to remind you of those times that you spent together.

Accomplishment Activities

The rationale for engaging in activities that give you a sense of accomplishment is similar to the rationale for engaging in pleasurable activities. It's easy to understand that you may not feel like engaging in goal-directed activities following a reproductive loss. However, after a period of not doing so, tasks that need your attention will pile up, leading you to feel overwhelmed on top of all of the other emotions that you are juggling. A pile-up of tasks is, of course, aversive for anyone, and it has the potential to propel the vicious cycle by making you feel more sad and depressed, which in turn fuels further avoidance behavior. Thus, doing one thing each day that gives you a sense of mastery or accomplishment will give you a moment in which your mood is improved and a sense that you are in control of something in your life.

What if it seems like there is so much to do that you don't know where to start? Perhaps the best activities to choose are ones that give you both pleasure and a sense of accomplishment. Activities that might fit this bill include gardening or cooking a favorite meal (which will also help you to reach the goal of eating regularly). Conversely, you might avoid activities that would give you a sense of accomplishment but that you find highly aversive. If there are nonessential things that you need to address as a result of the reproductive loss, you can put those off until you feel strong enough to deal with them.

STRATEGIES FOR GETTING BY

In addition to the self-care suggestions I have discussed to this point in the chapter, other strategies can help you get by in the first weeks following a reproductive loss or trauma. These strategies are particularly useful when you find yourself overcome by sadness, guilt, anxiety, anger, and so on because they give you the tiniest bit of pleasure or calm in the midst of emotional pain. They don't necessarily take the pain away, but they soften its edges so that you can endure it. They allow you to experience and accept the pain with as much grace and dignity as is possible in these circumstances. Thus, they are strategies that will help you to get through what seem to be unbearable moments.

Take a "Vacation"

I write "vacation" in quotation marks because it could refer to an actual vacation or a metaphorical vacation. It could be a weekend away with your partner to a soothing location (e.g., the beach, the mountains, a bed-and-breakfast). It could just be a day or part of a day when you take a vacation from the demands of your life, such as a shopping trip or a sporting event. It could even be a day that you devote to thinking of something else other than the loss or trauma, such as reading a book cover to cover or knitting an entire piece of clothing, or a part of the day when you use imagery to bring yourself to a calm, soothing place (e.g., the location of your annual family vacations, your favorite scenic destination).

In some ways, taking a "vacation" is an extension of the self-care strategy of engaging in a pleasurable activity. The idea is that it gives you something to look forward to and a change of scenery that has the potential to refresh and center you. Be careful, though, of taking a more "permanent vacation" from your grief and emotions doing things like stifling them, throwing yourself into an array of demanding activities, or using alcohol or drugs as an escape. "Permanent vacations" simply prolong avoidance of dealing with the loss or trauma. The "vacation" is meant to be a short-term strategy that will give you a brief reprieve from the emotional pain so that you are in a better position to deal with it when you return.

Distraction

What should you do if, no matter what, your mind keeps going back to the reproductive loss, and you desperately want it out of your head? It is tempting to try to suppress or squelch the thoughts—telling yourself that you are not allowed to go there. Unfortunately, research by the late Harvard professor Daniel Wegner showed that thought suppression does not work and that it, in fact, increases, rather than decreases, the frequency of unwanted thoughts. In his experiments, he instructed some of his research subjects to think about anything they wanted within a short period of time, with the exception of a white bear. As you might imagine, the research subjects who were told not to think of a white bear reported a much higher frequency of thoughts about the very thing they were not supposed to think about, relative to research subjects who were told that they could think about anything they wanted to think about, including white bears. The same thing happens when you are trying to suppress thoughts about more serious issues, such as a reproductive loss.

Instead, try to focus on something that will take all of your mental energy, like doing a crossword puzzle or Sudoku or putting together a jigsaw puzzle. In fact, you might want to have readily available a few things that can distract you from your thoughts so that you have access to these activities when you need them. Countless clients have told me that this advice is invaluable because when they are in a moment of extreme emotional distress, they have trouble remembering distractions that would be helpful. If you don't have access to something tangible that will facilitate distraction, try counting backward by threes. The idea is that by focusing your attention on a task that requires your full mental capacity, there won't be room to focus on thoughts of the loss or trauma.

Self-Soothing

Self-soothing is one of my favorite parts of a treatment approach that is in the family of cognitive behavioral therapies called *dialectical behavior therapy*. It is an approach for getting through the moment by doing things that fully engage one or more of the five senses in a pleasurable or soothing manner. Exhibit 2.2 contains a partial listing of ways to engage the five senses through self-soothing. These are not the only ways to gain the benefit of self-soothing; every person is unique and will find different things soothing. I encourage you to develop your own list of simple activities that you would find self-soothing and write them down on a piece of paper or an index card. Be sure you remember where you put the paper or card so that you can easily locate it in times of distress.

EXHIBIT 2.2. Self-Soothing Ideas

Vision

- View pieces of art at an art museum.
- Observe beautiful scenery in person, in a book, on television, or on the Internet.
- Watch the rain or snow fall.
- Arrange flowers in a bouquet and place them in a central location in your home.

Hearing

- Listen to pleasing or soothing music.
- Listen to recordings of nature sounds (e.g., ocean waves).
- Listen to church bells.
- Listen to the soft breeze.

Smell

- Light a scented candle or incense.
- Breathe in the smell of flowers.
- Smell freshly cut grass.
- Bake a pie or bread and take in the aroma.

Taste

- Savor one square of chocolate.
- Enjoy a soothing drink like herbal tea or hot cocoa.
- Pay close attention to the minty sensations of mouthwash.
- Slowly eat a special treat.

Touch

- Pet a dog or cat.
- Rub lotion on your arms and legs.
- Curl up in a warm, fuzzy blanket.
- Take a bubble bath.

Note. For additional suggestions, see Linehan (1993) and McKay, Wood, and Brantley (2007).

Controlled Breathing

The power of breathing is tremendous. The breath is a vehicle for you to connect to your inner core, and you can always rely on it, even in the midst of chaos. It serves as distraction in that it focuses your attention on the breath instead of your emotional distress. It also allows you to regulate your physical and mental states, so that it ramps down your response to stress or emotional upset and restores a sense of controllability and predictability.

One word of caution: Many people refer to *deep breathing* when they think of using their breath to manage emotional distress. Deep breathing refers to breathing through the diaphragm to fill your lungs fully with air, rather than in a shallow manner by moving your shoulders up and down. However, many people mistakenly believe that deep breathing means that they need to take in as much air as possible, especially if their stress or emotional upset is leaving them short of breath. Paradoxically, taking in as much air as possible has the potential to exacerbate your physiological symptoms of stress and emotional upset, not decrease them. This is so because when oxygen is taken in your body, it eventually converts to carbon dioxide. The body's marker for the degree to which one's breathing is regulated is the level of carbon dioxide. When the body detects that there is an excess of carbon dioxide, several physiological processes are activated. For example, the hemoglobin in the blood (i.e., the chemical that carries oxygen around the body) increases its "stickiness" for oxygen and does not allow it to be easily released. The blood vessels constrict, decreasing the likelihood that oxygen will get to your brain and to your extremities. When these things occur, you will probably experience many of the physiological symptoms that you are trying to manage, such as lightheadedness and dizziness because of the lack of oxygen going to the brain and tingling and numbness in your extremities because of the lack of oxygen that is able to travel there.

Thus, I recommend to my clients that they approach breathing exercises from a standpoint of regaining control, rather than from a standpoint of breathing deeply. Here is a simple *controlled breathing* protocol that you can use in times of emotional upset:

- Find a quiet, relaxing location, and dim the lights, if possible.
- Sit in a reclining position or lie on your back.
- Close your eyes if you are comfortable in doing so; otherwise, fix your gaze on one spot in the room.
- Breathe in through your mouth or nose to a count of 3 (1 – 2 – 3). Take a brief pause, and exhale through your mouth or nose to a count of 5 (1 – 2 – 3 – 4 – 5).
- Continue this practice for 10 breaths.
- Be sure to take in a normal amount of air in each breath.
- If you are lying down, check to make sure that your belly is moving up and down, as if a balloon is inflating and deflating. Your belly expanding and contracting in this manner is indicative of diaphragmatic breathing.
- Remain with your eyes closed until you are ready to open them.
- Assess what is different after going through this exercise. Taking the time to note the benefits of controlled breathing will increase the likelihood that you will use it in the future.

There are all sorts of breathing procedures that you can find in books and online, and as long as you are taking in the usual amount of air in each breath, the specifics don't matter. Many of my clients find that it is best to either (a) have a simple procedure (such as that just described) in your mind so that you need not read a protocol as you are trying to gain the benefits from controlled breathing or (b) listen to an audio file of a soothing voice that leads you through the exercise. Audio files can be purchased on CDs or as MP3 files on sites such as itunes.com and Amazon.com. These services typically allow you to listen to an excerpt of the file so that you can determine the file that is the most pleasing and helpful for you.

Muscle Relaxation

Like controlled breathing, *muscle relaxation* is a calming technique that focuses on one major physiological manifestation of distress— muscle tension. Moreover, many people practice combined muscle relaxation and controlled breathing, such that they focus on their breathing as they relax certain muscle groups. Also as with controlled breathing, there are many muscle relaxation protocols that can be found in books, CDs, and MP3 audio files.

My favorite muscle relaxation procedure is *progressive muscle relaxation*, which is the systematic tensing and relaxing of 16 muscle groups to achieve a state of calm. Many of my clients wonder why they are being instructed to tense their muscles if the purpose of the exercise is relaxation. My response is that if I simply told them to relax a muscle group, they would look at me like I am crazy. By tensing the particular muscle group, it allows one to observe the contrast with letting go of that tension and then relaxing. It also allows for a sensation of warmth to be experienced after one releases the tension.

Skill in muscle relaxation is best acquired when you practice at times when you are not particularly upset or distressed. It is a lot like learning how to play golf: It takes some time for you to become proficient and for your muscles to build up muscle memory. Thus, if you are a novice and try to use it when you are upset, you might not perceive that you get much benefit. Here is a simple muscle relaxation protocol that you can practice:

- Find a quiet, relaxing location, and dim the lights if possible.
- Sit in a reclined position or lie down on your back.
- Close your eyes if you are comfortable doing so; otherwise, fix your gaze on one spot in the room.

- Consider beginning the exercise with controlled breathing protocol such as the procedure I described earlier.
- Tense each major muscle group for 5 to 10 seconds and release the tension for 15 to 20 seconds. Major muscle groups include the feet, calves, thighs, abdominal region, hands and forearms, biceps, chest/shoulders/upper back area, neck and throat, lower cheeks and jaw, and upper cheeks and forehead.
- When you release the tension with each muscle group, exhale through your mouth or nose so that you can infuse your breath into the relaxation that you are experiencing.
- Keep your eyes closed until you are ready to open them.
- Assess what is different after going through this exercise. Taking the time to note the benefits of muscle relaxation will increase the likelihood that you will use it in the future.

Rather than try to follow written instructions, I recommend listening to an audio file when you do muscle relaxation. Many of my clients have told me that when they are trying to follow written instructions, their relaxation is continually being interrupted by having to pick up a piece of paper and read the next set of muscles to be tensed and relaxed. Moreover, many clients say that a soothing voice helps them to focus on the task at hand. If you choose not to use an audio file, I recommend that you tense and relax muscle groups in sequential order in terms of their location in your body. For example, I often start with my feet and work my way systematically up to my forehead. This simple procedure minimizes the amount of mental energy you spend deciding what muscle group to do next.

MAXIMIZING THE BENEFITS AND MINIMIZING THE OBSTACLES

Most people will say that, in theory, these strategies make sense. However, there is a big difference between understanding why these strategies work and actually using them. In this section, I describe some ways to maximize the success of these strategies and minimize the obstacles that can interfere with their use.

Reminder Phone Calls

When Kristin was 10 days' post–pregnancy loss, she had been spending most of her time in bed, either sleeping or watching reruns on television. She had taken only one shower in this 10-day period and had eaten only sporadically. Her partner was concerned but admitted that he was at a loss to know how to provide support. After he shared his concerns with Kristin's older sister, a licensed clinical social worker, the sister reached out to Kristin to help her to take steps toward resuming self-care. She called Kristin each the morning to encourage her to get out of bed, shower, and eat breakfast, and she helped Kristin to identify a plan for the manner in which she was spending her day to ensure that she was engaging in activities that were pleasurable and gave her a sense of accomplishment.

Not all people are fortunate enough to have a family member or friend who is a mental health professional. However, family members and friends who read this volume can serve as coaches as their loved one attempts to implement the strategies to get through painful moments. Like Kristin's sister, they can call their loved one to wake her up in the morning, helping to keep her on a regular sleep schedule and prepare for the day (that is, if the loved one agrees that it would be helpful to do so and not seem like punishment or pressure). They can also serve as soundboards as their loved one identifies one or more activities to do during the day that are associated with a sense of pleasure or accomplishment.

Implement Gradually

This chapter contains a large array of strategies and tools to take care of yourself and get by; individually, the systematic implementation of any one of them can make a small but meaningful difference. However, the collective viewing of these tools and strategies has the potential to leave you feeling overwhelmed. "What should I do first? It seems too much to go from sleeping all day to getting up at a regular time, preparing meals, exercising, and connecting with others." Here, the principles of problem solving that I describe in greater detail in Chapter 8 can be of use.

I have several suggestions for determining where to start. It could be that one of the self-care areas jumps out at you as being particularly problematic and that, by addressing it first, you expect to obtain a noticeable amount of relief. Thus, one approach could be to start with the area in which you predict that you would gain the most benefit. On the other hand, it could just as easily be the case that it seems too overwhelming to start with the most problematic area. Another approach, then, is to start with something manageable, implement some behavioral changes, and notice their effects on your mood and functioning. This approach has the potential to give you some confidence that you *can* manage your emotional distress, which increases the likelihood that you will tackle some of the other areas.

The idea here is to implement these skills gradually, rather than attempting to immediately plunge into an entirely new way of being. For example, with her sister's help, Kristin recognized that staying in bed most of the day was hurting her, rather than helping her, but it had quickly developed into a habit that she did not know how to break. Rather than starting with the expectation that she would only sleep 8 hours a day during the evening hours, she committed to a graduated plan that she implemented over the course of several days. For the first 3 days, she focused on getting up by noon and not sleeping again until 8 p.m. Then, she gradually shifted the time that she got out of bed in the morning, with a target of 8 a.m. She also gradually shifted the time at which she went to bed in the evening, with a target of 10 p.m. All the while, she identified some activities that she would do during waking hours so that she would not sleep out of boredom, despair, or hopelessness. The key is to remember that these changes do not need to occur overnight and that the effort that you put into self-care and getting by is just as important, if not more important, than the actual outcome.

Don't Expect Miracles

As I stated previously in the section on exercise, it is crucial to have realistic expectations for yourself and for the manner in which these self-care and getting-by strategies will affect your emotional distress. These tools and strategies might soften the pain, but they will not take it away. You will still have some bad days, and on occasion you might even reject these tools and strategies and stay in bed. Having a setback does not mean that you are a failure, nor does it mean that you are back at square one. It means that you are a human being who is struggling with a profound loss. On the other hand, when implemented systematically, these tools and strategies will very likely make a difference. Commit to them, see them through in their entirety, notice their positive effects when you experience them, and let go of the times when they do not seem to be helpful. And know that even if, in any one moment, you do not experience relief from your tremendous emotional distress, you are still doing something helpful for your mind and body.

NOTES ABOUT ONGOING MEDICAL CARE

Many readers who experienced a pregnancy loss will have to return to the obstetrician for a follow-up appointment in the weeks after the loss. It is understandable that going to the obstetrician's office is the last thing you would want to do; you may expect it to bring back many painful memories and emotions. As I mentioned in Chapter 1, it can be excruciating to be in the waiting room with so many other women who are visibly pregnant. *When you are making the appointment and again when you arrive, let the receptionist know about your recent loss or trauma.* Very often, they can find an alternative place where you can wait for your appointment, away from the other patients. You can also come prepared with other things to occupy your attention as you wait for your appointment, such as a compelling movie downloaded to your tablet device or a gripping novel.

In addition, you might have to endure even more procedures to determine the possible cause of the loss. For example, some women who have experienced pregnancy losses are asked to undergo a hysterosalpingography, commonly referred to as an HSG, to determine whether anything about the structure of the uterus and shape of the fallopian tubes is abnormal and could account for the recent pregnancy loss. This procedure can feel invasive, uncomfortable, and even a bit painful. It can evoke painful memories of the invasive procedures you had during fertility treatments or when you lost the baby. Plan in advance for these emotional experiences and "cope ahead." Do you need to engage in controlled breathing, muscle relaxation, or self-soothing before the procedure? Should you bring a supportive person from your social support network with you to the procedure? Or should you plan a "vacation" for after the procedure, such as a spa day or a drive through the country?

PREPARING FOR LONG-TERM EMOTIONAL CARE

Planning ahead can be helpful for circumstances other than ongoing medical care. For example, many readers will be preparing to go back to work, school, or volunteer work. Reengaging in these activities can bring a host of anxieties, such as how to share the news of the loss with acquaintances and how to handle sudden instances of sorrow and sadness. I encourage you to develop a personal self-care plan to consult when you resume your usual activities (see Figure 2.2). The

FIGURE 2.2. Personal Self-Care Plan

My Personal Self-Care Plan

This is what I will do to take care of myself as I resume my usual activities:

1.

2.

3.

4.

These are the triggers that I expect to experience as I resume my usual activities:

1.

2.

3.

4.

This is how I will handle the emotional distress associated with the triggers:

1.

2.

3.

4.

People I can call if I need support:

1.

2.

3.

personal self-care plan can contain many of the tools and strategies described in this chapter, as well as other coping skills that you have found useful at other times in your life. This approach to "coping ahead" can be invaluable because it is often difficult to identify a particular self-care tool in moments of acute distress.

It is also important to think about planning ahead toward longer term emotional care. Although the acute edge of emotional distress may gradually diminish over time, many people who have experienced reproductive loss indicate that they continue to experience great heartache, which takes a toll on their mood and quality of life. You will still have times of emotional upset associated with your loss or trauma, and all of the strategies described in this chapter will continue to be useful in getting you through those moments. However, in preparing for longer term emotional care, two pieces must be in place. First, your self-care habits must become routine, and second, you should engage in goal-directed activities that are meaningful and satisfying that are not directly tied to having children. In other words, you must ensure that the sole source of life satisfaction does not rest on having a child but that you have many gratifying parts of your life on which you can rely, independent from having a child (or having more children than you have at present). The next chapter describes ways to achieve these aims.

CHAPTER 3

GETTING INVOLVED IN LIFE IN THE LATER WEEKS

By now, several weeks have passed since your reproductive loss. Perhaps you have returned to work, resumed your volunteer work, gone back to school, or reengaged with other activities that were part of your usual routine. This is a terrific step in your healing journey—a regular routine will give you purpose and structure. Nevertheless, what was a satisfying routine before the loss or trauma might seem woefully inadequate now. Things have changed, and you may be wondering how you can possibly go back to normal. The people around you might seem to be going about their lives as if nothing has happened. Even though you might be going through the motions of resuming your normal routine, you might continue to be painfully aware of your recent loss or trauma. If you received a great deal of support and sympathy in the early weeks following the loss, it is likely that the pace of such gestures has slowed considerably.

You might be wondering when these experiences will go away, or conversely, whether they will persist indefinitely. Know that the intensity of these experiences will lessen over time, even if they get exacerbated in particular moments, such as a reminder of the loss or trauma. Moreover, they will be less consuming if you are living your life with as much quality and satisfaction as possible. Many of my clients talk about creating a *new normal* in light of the loss or trauma. This chapter discusses some ideas as you begin to create your new normal.

DOING WHAT YOU VALUE

In the previous chapter, I explained the importance of engaging in activities that are associated with a sense of pleasure or accomplishment, or both. The more of these activities you engage in, the greater will be the buffer against depression and other adverse emotional experiences. You will get positive reinforcement from your environment and minimize the degree to which your problems and other requirements of daily living overwhelm you. The technical term for this strategy is *behavioral activation*.

In the first weeks following a reproductive loss, behavioral activation usually consists of doing *any* activity that will give you even the slightest sense of pleasure or accomplishment. In many instances, these activities are straightforward and easy to implement because you won't have much energy and motivation to do a lot of planning and preparation. Those sorts of simple activities might include watching a movie, reading a book, or going for coffee with a friend.

Now, it is time to think about behavioral activation as systematically pursuing one or more interests or passions that will enhance your quality of life and life satisfaction. This means that you will live and make choices for how to spend your time according to the values that you hold dearest.

What Are My Values?

I view living a *value-driven life* as operating according to two dimensions: the roles that are most important to you (i.e., *what* you are doing with your time) and the kind of person you want to be (i.e., *how* you carry out those roles). Take a look at Figure 3.1. I propose

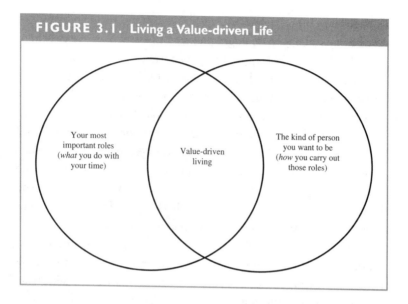

FIGURE 3.1. Living a Value-driven Life

Your most important roles (*what* you do with your time)

Value-driven living

The kind of person you want to be (*how* you carry out those roles)

that living a value-driven life occurs when the two dimensions intersect in the middle—that is, when you are engaging in the activities that are consistent with your most important roles, and you are enacting these activities according to the person you want to be.

It is not difficult to imagine that many readers of this book would say that the most important role to which they aspire is being a parent. If you have children, that is more than reasonable. The key in this scenario, though, is to focus your role on being a parent to the child or children that you have right now, rather than defining your role in terms of the number of children you hope to have. If you do not have children, you need not abandon being a parent as a role to which you aspire. However, I strongly encourage you to identify other roles you can assume *right now* that will be meaningful to you. I'd also encourage you to expand your view of parenting to one of being a part of a larger family. The rationale behind this is that you acknowledge that you are a valued member of a family and provide and receive family support even if you do not have children. This might include support to or from a sibling, parent, grandparent, niece, nephew, or godchild.

In Figure 3.2, I apply the pie-chart technique in a different manner than I did in Chapter 2. Here, I'm using the pie chart to illustrate how important roles make up our identities, or the manner in which we view ourselves. It's very possible that becoming a parent has dominated your personal pie chart. The top part of Figure 3.2 is an extreme example of that; the person depicted in this pie chart viewed becoming a parent as her only important role. When she was in danger of losing that role following a pregnancy loss, she had no other pieces of the pie on which to rely, and she had no other avenues for obtaining pleasure, gratification, and meaning.

The bottom part of Figure 3.2 depicts a more balanced conceptualization of one's important roles. After her pregnancy loss, the person represented in this pie chart by no means viewed her life as complete. In fact, although she tried to view becoming a parent as but one part of being a valued wife and family member, she viewed that piece of the pie, for the most part, as disappointing. However, she had other roles that she considered as important parts of who she is. She took pride in being a successful professional in her role as physical therapist at the largest hospital in the city. She was a runner who regularly competed in 10K and half-marathon races. She thrived on traveling, whether it was to weekend destinations that were only an hour or two away from her home or her yearly adventure travel vacation. Furthermore, she was just learning to play the acoustic guitar and beginning to see music as playing a greater and greater part of her life. Viewed in this manner, her pregnancy loss contributed to 25% of her pie chart as being disappointing, but she had 75% intact. That 75% helped her through the later weeks following her pregnancy loss by giving her the sense that she had a rich, meaningful existence. My wish for you is that you can conceptualize your own pie chart with your most important roles that contribute

FIGURE 3.2. Roles Pie Chart: Sample

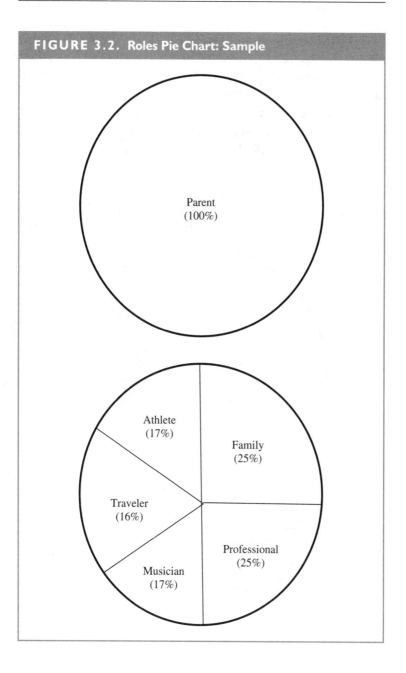

to a sense of meaning or value in your life; acknowledge the pieces of the pie that are going well; attend to the pieces that you can engage right now, regardless of whether you are a parent, and, if needed, nurture and cultivate new pieces that have the potential to provide meaning and satisfaction. Figure 3.3 gives you space to do this.

The important roles are just one part of the equation; as Figure 3.1 suggests, the *how* of implementing the roles is just as

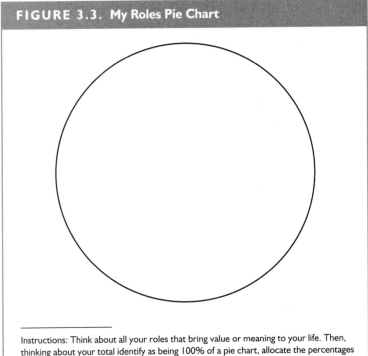

FIGURE 3.3. My Roles Pie Chart

Instructions: Think about all your roles that bring value or meaning to your life. Then, thinking about your total identify as being 100% of a pie chart, allocate the percentages that each role contributes to your identity. Draw the pieces of the pie in the pie chart below, roughly equivalent to the percentage to which you allocated each one of your roles. Label each piece of the pie and its corresponding percentage that contributes to your identity.

important to consider as you live a value-driven life. Even if you are engaging in fairly mundane activities, acting according to these values will help you to maximize the amount of satisfaction you can get from them. It can be satisfying, in and of itself, to behave according to the person you want to be. Many people have never before considered these values and have a hard time narrowing down the person they want to be. Take a look at Exhibit 3.1 and choose the five characteristics that align most closely to the person you want to be. Then think about ways you can live your life according to these characteristics, whether you are engaging in activities associated with your most important roles, or whether you are engaging in mundane activities.

EXHIBIT 3.1. The Person You Want to Be

Loving	Accomplished	Loyal	Honest
Loved by others	Professional	Hardworking	Spiritual
Nurturing	Persistent	Caring	Friendly
Encouraging	Community-minded	Athletic	Musical
Artistic	Effective	Centered	Thoughtful
Mindful	Influential	Respected	Focused
Creative	Wise	Well-rounded	Articulate
Interesting	Unique	Efficient	Strong
Unwavering	Physically fit	Connected with others	Autonomous
Sensitive toward others	Flexible	Active	Responsible
Engaged	Well-read	Family-oriented	Diligent

How Am I Currently Spending My Time?

Living a value-driven life can seem like a tall order when one is not feeling well. Where do you start? The place where cognitive behavioral therapists start with their clients is to get a sense of how, currently, they are spending their time, as well as the manner in which the activities that fill their time are associated with a sense of pleasure and accomplishment and are consistent with their values.

Thus, I encourage you to commit to a 3-day period of recording the manner in which you are spending your time. This exercise is called *activity monitoring*. Be sure to choose days that reflect your typical schedule. It is often helpful to include one weekend day because many people find that they engage in the most pleasurable and enjoyable activities during the weekends. For each activity that you record, rate three things: (a) a "P" rating for the amount of pleasure you got from the activity (0 = *no pleasure*, 10 = *the most pleasure possible*), (b) an "A" rating for the amount of accomplishment you sensed from the activity (0 = *no accomplishment*, 10 = *the most accomplishment possible*), and (c) a "V" rating for the degree to which your engagement in the activities was consistent with your values (0 = *inconsistent with values*, 10 = *very consistent with values*). Then, at the end of each day, make an overall rating of your mood (0 = *worst mood you've ever experienced*, 10 = *best mood you've ever experienced*). Figure 3.4 is a sample of activity monitoring exercise for Amelia, who experienced a reproductive loss approximately 3 months before completing the exercise, and Figure 3.5 is a blank activity log for you to write in your own activities; the times in which you are doing them; the amount of accomplishment, pleasure, and value you get from your activities; and your overall mood.

The purpose of this activity is to draw specific conclusions about the degree to which you are living a valued life. Let's first take a look at Amelia's activity monitoring exercise. What do you notice?

FIGURE 3.4. Amelia's Activity Monitoring Exercise

Day and date: Friday, September 28, 2012	
7 a.m.–8 a.m.: Woke up, morning routine	P = 2; A = 2; V = 0
8 a.m.–8:30 a.m.: Morning commute	P = 0; A = 1; V = 2
8:30 a.m.–9:30 a.m.: Team meeting at work	P = 3; A = 4; V = 4
9:30–11 a.m.: Completed report	P = 3; A = 9; V = 7
11 a.m.–12 p.m.: Calls to clients	P = 3; A = 6; V = 6
12 p.m.–12:30 p.m.: Lunch break with coworkers	P = 8; A = 3; V = 8
12:30–1 p.m.: Meeting with supervisor	P = 2; A = 6; V = 7
1 p.m.–3 p.m.: Research for next project	P = 4; A = 9; V = 8
3 p.m.–4 p.m.: New employee training	P = 4; A = 7; V = 6
4 p.m.–5 p.m.: Planning for next week's business travel	P = 3; A = 4; V = 5
5 p.m.–5:30 p.m.: Evening commute	P = 0; A = 1; V = 2
5:30 p.m.–6 p.m.: Unwind, TV in background	P = 1; A = 0; V = 1
6 p.m.–6:30 p.m.: Prepare dinner	P = 2; A = 2; V = 4
6:30 p.m.–7:30 p.m.: Eat dinner	P = 4; A = 0; V = 6
7:30 p.m.–8 p.m.: Walk dog with husband	P = 4; A = 4; V = 7
8 p.m.–10:30 p.m.: TV	P = 3; A = 0; V = 1
10:30 p.m.: Bedtime	P = 2; A = 0; V = 5
Overall mood for the day:	3

Note. P = pleasure; A = accomplishment; V = values.

First, her mood is quite low—a 3 out of 10. The main activities in which she engaged during the day were work, domestic activities (i.e., preparing and eating dinner, walking the dog), and watching TV. She reported a low sense of pleasure, accomplishment, and value in the activities in which she engaged in the early morning

FIGURE 3.5. Blank Activity Log

Day and date:	
	P = ; A = ; V =
	P = ; A = ; V =
	P = ; A = ; V =
	P = ; A = ; V =
	P = ; A = ; V =
	P = ; A = ; V =
	P = ; A = ; V =
	P = ; A = ; V =
	P = ; A = ; V =
	P = ; A = ; V =
	P = ; A = ; V =
	P = ; A = ; V =
	P = ; A = ; V =
	P = ; A = ; V =
	P = ; A = ; V =
	P = ; A = ; V =
	P = ; A = ; V =
	P = ; A = ; V =
Overall mood for the day:	
Day and date:	
	P = ; A = ; V =
	P = ; A = ; V =
	P = ; A = ; V =
	P = ; A = ; V =
	P = ; A = ; V =
	P = ; A = ; V =
	P = ; A = ; V =
	P = ; A = ; V =
	P = ; A = ; V =
	P = ; A = ; V =

FIGURE 3.5. Blank Activity Log (Continued)

	P = ; A = ; V =
	P = ; A = ; V =
	P = ; A = ; V =
	P = ; A = ; V =
	P = ; A = ; V =
	P = ; A = ; V =
	P = ; A = ; V =
	P = ; A = ; V =
Overall mood for the day:	
Day and date:	
	P = ; A = ; V =
	P = ; A = ; V =
	P = ; A = ; V =
	P = ; A = ; V =
	P = ; A = ; V =
	P = ; A = ; V =
	P = ; A = ; V =
	P = ; A = ; V =
	P = ; A = ; V =
	P = ; A = ; V =
	P = ; A = ; V =
	P = ; A = ; V =
	P = ; A = ; V =
	P = ; A = ; V =
	P = ; A = ; V =
	P = ; A = ; V =
Overall mood for the day:	

Note. P = pleasure; A = accomplishment; V = values.

(e.g., her morning routine, her morning commute). These ratings did not surprise Amelia; she often dreaded getting out of bed and going in to work. Although her activities at work did not bring a great deal of pleasure, many of them brought her a sense of accomplishment. A notable exception was her half hour lunch break, which she spent with colleagues. Not only was that lunch pleasurable, it was also rated as being highly consistent with her values because she viewed herself as a good friend and listener toward others. She also rated many of her work activities as being highly consistent with her values because she took pride in being a hard worker and believed that she was making a meaningful contribution to the company, even though at times some of her work activities were unpleasant (e.g., a meeting with her supervisor).

Notice how Amelia spent her time after work. After she returned home from her commute, she spent some unstructured time unwinding and watching TV, then engaging in domestic activities with her husband, and then spending the remainder of the evening watching TV. You might have observed that none of her pleasure or accomplishment ratings were higher than 4, although she regarded eating dinner and walking the dog with her husband as being consistent with her value of spending quality time with her husband. Amelia was a bit surprised when she evaluated the ratings she had made. She had always assumed that watching TV at night was an activity that would help her relax and unwind; however, her ratings suggested that she got little pleasure or accomplishment from this activity, and she realized that watching TV was inconsistent with her values of being active and engaged in life.

According to behavioral theories of depression, participating in activities associated with pleasure, accomplishment, and value should be associated with a positive change in mood. The goal, then, of doing activity monitoring is to identify places in which you can work in activities associated with a greater sense of pleasure, accomplishment, and value than you are currently. Amelia drew three conclusions from her activity monitoring exercise. First, the early morning was particularly difficult for her, and the mundane activities in which she typically engaged in the morning were not helping her mood. Second, although she got a sense of accomplishment and value when she was at work, other than at lunch, she derived little pleasure. Third, she was getting less pleasure, accomplishment, and value from her evening activities than was desired. She also realized that she was not engaging in optimal self-care (e.g., not taking off her makeup and washing her face before going to bed, falling asleep in her work clothes).

Take some time now to draw your own conclusions from your activity monitoring exercise. How are the activities in which you are engaging associated with your overall mood? Where are places that you can work in more activities associated with pleasure, a sense of accomplishment, or a sense of value? Are there particular times of the day where you struggle and need to focus on ways to take care of yourself? The following section provides specific guidance on what you can do with this information.

How Can I Live More Consistently With My Values?

On the basis of the activity monitoring exercise, you can begin to work in activities that give you a sense of pleasure, accomplishment, and value. Cognitive behavioral therapists call this *activity scheduling*. The idea behind activity scheduling is that you use the activity monitoring exercise to identify times that are particularly devoid of activities associated with pleasure, accomplishment, or value, as Amelia did, and then schedule in additional activities that would achieve these aims. For example, to address the dearth of meaningful early morning activities, which Amelia suspected contributed to her dread and overall malaise in the mornings, she and her husband decided to get up a half hour early in the morning, sit at the kitchen table together while reading the paper, and drink a special blend of coffee. They began to make the choosing of coffee flavors into a game, choosing a new one each week when they went grocery shopping and rating its flavor once they tried it. To address the dearth of pleasurable activities while at work, Amelia scheduled two brief activities that were pleasurable but would not interfere with her responsibilities. In the mornings around 10 a.m., she decided that she would have a nutritious snack of yogurt and nuts that she prepared at home, eating them mindfully without multitasking at the computer or on the phone. In the afternoons around 2:30 p.m., she and her favorite coworker decided to take a break and go on a 15-minute "power walk" outdoors around the premises of the building. Amelia was particularly pleased with these additions because they were also consistent with her values of being a good friend and being healthy and active.

After completing the activity monitoring exercise, Amelia realized that she needed to shift her evening activities away from mundane activities and watching TV. She also found it curious that, although she valued spending time with her husband eating their dinner and walking their dog, she did not get much pleasure and accomplishment out of doing these activities. On the basis of this information, Amelia made three changes. First, she decided to break out of the habit of cooking the same meals over and over and to challenge herself to try some new recipes. Not only did she anticipate that this change would increase her sense of pleasure, accomplishment, and value when she was preparing dinner, she also suspected it would be a topic of lively discussion with her husband during dinner and that they could spend time together planning additional meals for the remainder of the week. Second, Amelia expanded the time spent outside with the dog, such that at times she and her husband took longer, more scenic routes, and at other times they played with the dog in the yard before going inside. Third, Amelia expanded the repertoire of activities in which she engaged in the evening before going to bed. She opted to retain 1 hour of TV time most nights because there were shows that she found appealing. However, she identified several other activities that would bring her pleasure and, at times, a sense of accomplishment, such as participating in an adult education course once a week, scheduling phone dates with her high school and college friends who lived out of the area, and reading modern literature.

Amelia continued to track her activities and her mood for 2 more weeks to determine whether her new schedule made a difference in her life. She was pleased to see that her mood ratings had gradually risen from a level of 3 to levels of 6 to 8. She attributed this improvement in mood to having meaningful activities to which she could look forward and increased social contact with her friends, which had always been important to her. Although she did not know what her reproductive future held, she was comforted by the facts that she had strong relationships with her husband and friends and that she was developing a passion for cooking and creative writing.

Now it's your turn to schedule some activities on the basis of the conclusions that you drew from activity monitoring. Figure 3.6 is a worksheet that will help you accomplish this. In each row, record one activity that you will attempt to work into your schedule. In addition, identify a time that you will commit to engaging in the activity. Finally, assign a "P" if you expect that the activity will give you a sense of pleasure; an "A" if you expect that the activity will give you a sense of accomplishment; and a "V" if you expect that the activity will give you a sense of value. Many people find that they experience a combination of pleasure, accomplishment, and value from their activities, so it is OK to assign more than one letter. The reason for assigning these letters is so that you remember the ratio-

FIGURE 3.6. My Activity Schedule

Activity	When will I commit to doing this activity?	P, A, V

P = pleasure. A = accomplishment. V = values.

nale for scheduling the activity because that rationale will give you a clear sense of the pathway through which engaging in that activity will have a positive effect on your mood.

From my years of experience as a cognitive behavioral therapist, I have several tips that have the potential to increase the likelihood that activity scheduling will achieve its desired effect. They are as follows.

Give yourself a window of time for each activity. It's easy to become discouraged if you schedule an activity for, say, 2 p.m. on a Tuesday afternoon, and 2 p.m. comes, and something gets in the way of following through. When this happens, many people fall into an "all-or-nothing" thinking trap (see Chapters 4 and 5 for more description about this pattern of thinking), such that they say to themselves, "What's the point of doing any of the other activities that are scheduled? I already missed my first one!" I would encourage you, when you are scheduling activities, to balance specificity with flexibility. In other words, it is important to be specific enough in your scheduling to hold yourself accountable. Just saying to yourself, "I will go to the gym three times in the next week," does not provide enough clarification of when that might happen. On the other hand, narrowing down an activity to a precise hour might be too rigid because it does not account for the unexpected happenings that invariably occur in life. Thus, I often encourage people to schedule activities in broader time frames, such as *Tuesday afternoon* or *Friday night*. And, if even with this flexible scheduling you still miss an activity, it is OK. It takes time to shift your routine and develop new habits. Also, give yourself credit for the activities that you *do* complete. You have gone through a difficult, and even traumatic, experience recently, and you are allowed to give yourself permission to be less than perfect.

Have a backup plan. For the same reasons as I discussed previously, it is also wise to have a backup plan. The backup plan can consist of a completely different day and time frame in which to do the activity, or it can consist of a different activity you can do in the time frame that you had already reserved. Having a backup plan is especially important for activities that depend on good weather. For example, if you planned to go for a run on Tuesday afternoon, and it is raining, you can either go for a run on Wednesday afternoon, or you can exercise indoors by going to a Pilates class at the local gym, for example. As with scheduling events in broad time frames, having a backup plan gives you flexibility if something interferes with doing the activity that is scheduled, and it guards against discouragement and all-or-nothing thinking if you are unable to engage in the original activity that is scheduled.

Have a pool of activities from which you can choose. Many people prefer to reserve time, in general, for a meaningful activity, rather than scheduling in a specific activity several days in advance. This approach to activity scheduling reinforces flexibility and allows people to match their activity with the constraints of the moment. Let's consider a person who reserved a block of time on Saturday afternoons to engage in a meaningful activity. When the weather is good and she is feeling physically well, she might go on a hike. However, when she suspects that she is coming down with a cold, she might engage in a lower key but nevertheless pleasurable activity, such as curling up in front of the fire with a mystery that she has been looking forward to reading. This is the strategy that Amelia used for her weekday evenings. One night a week, she took a creative writing class. Aside from that night, on some evenings, she scheduled phone dates with her long-distance friends. On other evenings, she decided to read. Occasionally, she would complete assignments for her creative writing class.

Be reasonable. When you're trying to shift your routine, it is tempting to bite off more than you can chew. How many people do you know who, when they commit to regular exercise, decide that they are going to exercise 6 days a week, only to become discouraged after a couple of days and abandon their goal? Remember, you're still recovering from a devastating life event. You might consider starting small, only incorporating a couple of changes into your routine and monitoring the manner in which they affect your mood. As your mood begins to improve, you can work in more and more activities that are consistent with your values.

WHEN IT'S HARD TO GET STARTED

When you're recovering from a reproductive loss, much of what I've written in this chapter can seem easier said than done. I and many of my clients have been there. In this section, I describe some obstacles to behavioral activation and ways to overcome them.

It's too hard to do activities—I just don't have it in me. This reaction is understandable in light of the fact that you're not yet back to 100%. On the one hand, it's important to have reasonable expectations for what you can and can't do so that you don't set yourself up for disappointment. On the other hand, research by psychologist Sona Dimidjian and her colleagues clearly demonstrates that behavioral activation is a key component in overcoming depression. If you perceive that it's too hard to initiate activities, you might take the approach described in Chapter 2, such that you engage in one simple pleasurable activity and one simple accomplishment activity until you feel better. Another option is to jot down activities that you used to have in your routine—the ones that gave you a sense of pleasure, accomplishment, and value—and rate on a scale of 0 to 10 how difficult they are to do (e.g., 0 = *no difficulty*, 10 = *the most difficulty you can imagine*). Then work on implementing just the activities that have low ratings (e.g., 0, 1, or 2) and work up to the activities that are associated with more difficulty. A third option is to enlist people in your social support network. Perhaps someone in your social support network would be willing to take the lead in planning on activity, and you could participate once the details are worked out.

I don't know which activities to choose. Loss, trauma, grieving, and depression can serve as blinders that prevent you from considering the full range of potentially meaningful activities that are available to you. It's almost as if you have tunnel vision, being unable to see anything other than typical routine and habits by which you live your life. If you're having trouble identifying value-driven activities, ask yourself the following questions:

- What activities are most consistent with my values?
- In the past, what activities did I find meaningful and valuable?
- In the past, what activities enhanced my quality of life and life satisfaction?
- What are my skills and interests?
- What types of activities have I always wanted to try but never got around to pursuing?
- Who is a centered, well-adjusted person whom I admire? What are the kinds of activities in which that person typically engages?
- What are the kinds of activities in which my family members and friends engage? Can I join them to try out those activities?

These questions were what prompted Amelia to take the once-a-week creative writing class. She had always wanted to write short stories, but whenever she sat down to do so, she experienced "writer's block" because she doubted her writing ability. She often contemplated taking a creative writing course to learn some skills and boost her confidence level, but it always seemed like "life got in the way" when she had the opportunity to sign up for one (e.g., she was working long hours at work; it was winter, and she preferred to spending her evenings cozied up at home; she didn't want to spend the money at the moment). After her reproductive loss, she began to ask herself, "If not now, when?" She viewed creative writing as an outlet to channel her grief, to focus on developing a valued skill, and to cultivate a passion that she could have with her for the rest of her life no matter what happened.

Even after contemplating the answers to these questions, some people still have difficulty identifying activities that have the poten-

---

EXHIBIT 3.2. Examples of Value-Driven Activities

- Take martial arts classes.
- Learn a new craft (e.g., crocheting, knitting).
- Use your existing crafting knowledge and make a project.
- Train for a race.
- Volunteer at a soup kitchen.
- Volunteer at an animal shelter.
- Attend live music performances.
- Plant a garden.
- Redecorate a room in your house.
- Complete a home maintenance project.
- Write a short story.
- Travel to visit family or friends.
- Join a book club.
- Become a member of a local museum.
- Take horseback riding lessons.
- Learn to play a musical instrument.
- Join a bowling league.

---

tial to provide a sense of meaning and value. Exhibit 3.2 provides a sampling of some ideas. Note that these are not one-time activities; rather, these are interests, hobbies, and passions that can be pursued over time. The idea here is not to overwhelm you or pressure you into making a commitment for which you are not ready. Rather, the idea is to build additional pieces of your pie chart (see Figure 3.1, bottom part) so that if you must be going through reproductive challenges, you will have other sources of meaning and gratification in your life regardless of the number of children you have. You will expand your identity from one that is focused mainly on becoming a parent to one that reflects a centered, well-rounded individual who is talented and engaged.

SEIZE THE MOMENT

Even if you have difficulty identifying valued activities to pursue on a regular basis, chances are that opportunities will come your way that you did not expect or plan for. Perhaps a musical is coming through town and will play at a local theater. Perhaps a friend approaches you and asks you to take a Saturday morning beading class. Perhaps your pastor at church is implementing a new adult spiritual education class. I encourage you to embrace these opportunities that arise in your everyday life, even if you don't feel like it. Life has a way of being serendipitous, and it could very well turn out that an opportunity you pursue simply as a way of being more engaged in your life turns into a passion, gives you wisdom or insight that you would not otherwise have gotten, or allows you to meet people who significantly enhance your life. You very well might be struggling with a void or a sense of emptiness. Although no one would say that these activities would fill a void created by the loss of a child or an opportunity for a child, they do give you something valuable.

PUTTING IT ALL TOGETHER

You might be wondering: "How is this going to address my heartache? Isn't this just a way of avoiding the real issue—that I need to figure out how to get the family that I have always dreamed about having?" It's not reasonable to expect the heartache to be eliminated. Going through this experience has changed your life. However, the strategies described in this chapter are those that promote *engagement* in meaningful activities in your life, rather than *avoidance* of them. Approaching life in this manner will help you to manage your mood and attain a sense of centeredness that you likely will not have attain had you isolated yourself following the loss or trauma or had you become so consumed by it that you have no other avenues for joy and meaning in your life. Moreover, you are diversifying your sources of joy and meaning so that if you experience a disappointment (or even a devastating loss) in one area, you will have other well-developed areas to carry you through. It is also likely that by using the strategies described in this chapter, you will be in a better place to plan your reproductive future when you are in a position to do so.

I often think about the fact that, at the end of my life, I will want to look back and say, with confidence and zest, that it was a life well lived. There will be challenges, setbacks, and disappointments. There will be times when we doubt ourselves, have regrets, and wish things could be different. However, you have the power to create a well-lived life, regardless of the number of children you have. Right now, it doesn't feel like that is possible. The strategies described in this chapter will help you to take steps to overcome the emptiness after a reproductive loss or trauma one step at a time. They key is, in each moment when you are faced with a decision about how to spend your time, ask yourself, "Am I making a choice that is consistent with my values?"

CHAPTER 4

COPING WITH DISTURBING THOUGHTS AND IMAGES OF THE LOSS

So far, we have considered what you might do, *behaviorally*, to take care of yourself and get through your recent pregnancy loss or reproductive trauma. However, there is an equally important dimension to address in dealing with reproductive loss—the *cognitive* dimension. *Cognition* refers to thought, which includes perception, interpretation, reasoning, judgment, and memory. Cognition and behavior have reciprocal effects on one another. For example, if you are focused on how awful life is, then it is easy to isolate yourself or stay in bed. Conversely, if you are isolating yourself or staying in bed, it reinforces the notion that life is awful. This is an example of the manner in which the cognition–behavior cycle can work against you. Keep in mind, though, that just as the cognition–behavior cycle can work against you, it can also work for you. This and the next chapter will begin to show you how to do that.

Many people who have experienced a pregnancy loss fall into the trap of ruminating excessively about the past. They are often plagued by "what if" questions (e.g., "What if I caused this by doing _____?"), and they second-guess the choices they made that they perceive are related to the pregnancy. In addition, some people who have experienced pregnancy loss report intrusive images of the actual events surrounding the loss (e.g., going into preterm labor). These are examples of cognitions that are quite normal but that if left unchecked have the potential to interfere with behavioral activation and keep you mired in your emotional distress.

In this chapter, I help you identify common traps into which your thinking might fall, and I and provide specific suggestions for getting distance and perspective on these patterns of thinking. I also describe how you can apply a process called *thought modification* to manage these cognitions. Thought modification involves a set of skills that help you to identify distressing thoughts and images; evaluate the degree to which they are accurate, helpful, and adaptive; and, if necessary, modify these cognitions to be more accurate, helpful, and adaptive. The idea is that thinking in the most accurate, helpful, and adaptive manner will ensure that you are not experiencing more emotional upset than you have under the circumstances.

I am not suggesting that you "turn the other cheek" or put on a pair of "rose-colored glasses." There is no getting around the fact that what you experienced was awful. It is important to acknowledge honestly the myriad negatives associated with reproductive loss. However, I have found that it is easy to have tunnel vision for these negatives, such that one exclusively focuses on the worst parts of the experience at the expense of other pieces of information that might be helpful to acknowledge in making sense of the experience in its totality. Thought modification gives you the opportunity to identify these other pieces of information and make sure that you don't forget them when you are thinking about your recent loss or trauma.

COMMON TRAPS

Many clients who have gone through cognitive behavioral therapy (CBT) are educated about *cognitive distortions*, or patterns of thinking that are inaccurate and that perpetuate emotional distress because they are overly focused on the negative aspect of the situation at the expense of more neutral aspects. I call these cognitive distortions *traps*. When one thinks of a trap, an array of implications and images comes to mind. Traps keep people stuck. Traps interfere with the attainment of important goals. People who have fallen into traps often view themselves as helpless and powerless, which in turn can create a sense of hopelessness about the future. The traps that I describe in this section serve the same function because they have the potential to keep you stuck in a cycle of never-ending grief, preventing you from making meaning of your recent life circumstances. Here, I describe some of the traps into which people who have experienced reproductive loss often fall when they are fixated on their recent loss or infertility.

Personalization

Personalization refers to the process of taking excessive personal responsibility for the outcome of a situation, ignoring other factors that contributed to it or assigning excessive blame to ourselves even if the outcome was unavoidable. As you might surmise, many people who have endured a reproductive loss believe that it is their fault that the loss or trauma occurred. Some women question whether eating something forbidden might have caused a pregnancy loss; other women wonder whether a previous abortion or a sexually transmitted disease prevented them from getting pregnant or carrying a child to term. In fact, some people who perceive themselves as having sordid histories in which they have done things wrong believe that pregnancy loss or infertility is a punishment for past transgressions. In cases in which people who have experienced reproductive loss have an identifiable problem that they could not possibly control (e.g., low sperm count, problems with clotting), they nevertheless believe that it is their fault that the loss or trauma occurred—that they are its sole cause. The effect of personalization is that the person carries a tremendous amount of guilt and shame, perhaps affecting the degree to which she views herself as a good person or as a person of worth.

Labeling

A trap that often goes along with personalization is *labeling*, or the tendency to judge oneself in overly rigid and harsh terms. Some people who have experienced reproductive loss label themselves as defective, failures, or losers. These are examples of all-or-nothing thinking that prevents people from acknowledging their many strengths and accomplishments that would counteract the ideas that they are defective, failures, and losers. When people make such harsh judgments of themselves, it is not surprising that they would feel down, disempowered, and helpless. Such labels also provide a context for negative and unhelpful comparisons with others because it is easy to conclude that women who seemingly had children without difficulty have much more going for them than you do. One of my clients carried the belief that she was "less of a woman" than her peers who had children because she struggled with both pregnancy loss and infertility. Although she was highly successful and respected in her professional life, this label was so salient in her mind that it was activated every time she encountered a woman who had children.

Should Statements

Should statements are proclamations about the way things should be or should have turned out. They set high, rigid standards and expectations that fail to account for the curveballs life throws, setting up those who harbor these beliefs for disappointment and despair. Many perinatal women believe that they or their medical team should have done something differently for the baby to have lived or for a pregnancy to have occurred. Or, quite simply, they believe that this shouldn't have happened, that childbearing should not be this complicated. In theory, most of us would agree with these *should* statements. It would be wonderful if childbearing were not so difficult for many couples. However, excessive focus on these *should* statements prevents people from accepting that there are many risks in life and that things do not go as planned, which in turn perpetuates emotional distress.

Mind Reading

Mind reading occurs when we conclude that we know what another thinks, such as one's opinion of us, one's reaction to us, or reasons one behaves as he or she does. The problem with mind reading is that these thoughts are assumptions, but we take them as fact, usually without checking them out with the other person. Subsequently, we feel awkward in the presence of the other person, and we might make decisions that we later regret, such as avoiding her or him. Mind reading in people who have experienced a reproductive loss often centers on concerns that (a) others will pity them, (b) others believe that something is wrong with them or that they are defective, and (c) others think that they should "get over it."

Emotional Reasoning

Emotional reasoning refers to instances in which we conclude that things are awful and that they will not work because we are feeling so badly in the moment. There is no question that you will be experiencing an array of distressing emotions for many, many weeks following a reproductive loss. As much as is possible, it is important for you to be present with those emotions without arbitrarily extending the implications of them to other aspects of your life or to your future. Know that feeling badly right now does not necessarily mean that everything in your life is, and will be, forever horrible. And know that just because you are feeling badly right now does not necessarily mean you will have another loss and will be unable to get pregnant again.

Arbitrary Inference

Arbitrary inference refers to instances in which we establish an association between two things, when, in fact, they have no actual relation, and the presence of one does not at all determine the presence of the other. Sometimes arbitrary inference goes along with personalization. For example, if a woman believes that she is personally responsible for the loss of her child, she might conclude in no uncertain terms that the glass of red wine she drank absolutely caused the pregnancy loss. In reality, it is nearly impossible to draw a one-to-one correspondence from a specific maternal behavior and a pregnancy loss. When arbitrary inference manifests in this manner, it can be helpful to verify it with your obstetrician, who will almost certainly tell you that the behavior about which you are concerned did not cause the pregnancy loss.

Arbitrary inference also occurs when people who have experienced reproductive loss believe that because others have not experienced a pregnancy loss or had difficulty conceiving, their lives are somehow more fulfilling. The fact that another person has not experienced a reproductive loss does not automatically mean that her life his perfect. Although reproductive loss does indeed affect one's perception of fulfillment for some time after the event, it does not have to be equivalent to a lack of fulfillment forever, nor does it have to be equivalent to having a less fulfilling life than others. The application of the tools for living a valued life, described in Chapter 3, is one way to refute this idea.

STEPS TO THOUGHT MODIFICATION

If you're thinking that every single one of these traps characterizes you, you are not alone. In fact, to some degree, the traps characterize many of us much of the time, as we are taking in so much information in any one moment that we have to take shortcuts to process it all. When you are experiencing a period of emotional upset, however, the direction of the shortcuts inherent in the traps is usually geared toward the negative. In this section, I describe a tried-and-true procedure for recognizing and addressing patterns of thinking that have the potential to make you feel worse.

Identifying Distressing Thoughts and Images

The first step in thought modification is to identify the thoughts and images that are most distressing to you. In this chapter, we focus on distressing thoughts about the loss or trauma experience in and of itself, as well as its immediate aftermath; in the next chapter, we'll focus on distressing thoughts and images about the longer term and even distant future. Notice that I've been referring to *thoughts and images* throughout the chapter. Although many people experience distressing cognition in the form of verbal thoughts, some people think in pictorial form, such as an unwanted memory from the past. As you read this chapter and attempt the exercises, if you are having trouble identifying your thoughts, ask yourself whether you are experiencing any mental images or memories that are exacerbating your emotional distress.

The idea is to figure out what is running through your mind in times when you notice that you are particularly upset. The most basic question you can ask yourself is, "What was just running through my mind?" In many instances, your thoughts will remind you of some of the traps described earlier in this chapter. By slowing down and identifying what was running through your mind, you'll be able to link your thinking, or cognition, with the intensity of your emotional distress. You'll be able to see that the trap into which you're falling is likely exacerbating your emotional distress.

One way to keep track of your thoughts is to record them on something cognitive behavioral therapists call a *three-column thought record* (see Figure 4.1). The thought record is a tool that

Situation	Thought	Emotion and Intensity (0 = lowest intensity; 10 = highest intensity)

FIGURE 4.1. Three-Column Thought Record

organizes your distressing thoughts and clearly demonstrates the link between your cognition and your emotion that is triggered in specific situations. You can even write down the trap into which you're falling if it would be helpful for you to recognize that. It is best to record the situation, thought, and emotion as close to the moment as possible when you experience emotional distress to capture the experience as accurately and as powerfully as is possible. Although it can be a hassle to keep a thought record, doing so over the course of at least a few days will provide valuable information about the nature and frequency of thoughts that ultimately make you feel worse. You don't have to use the thought record format— any format will do as long as you record the situation, thought, and emotion. Some people keep notes in their smartphones. Other people prefer to create electronic files, such as a Microsoft Excel spreadsheet. Still others have found applications for their smartphones and tablets that provide an easy-access format to record thoughts (e.g., MoodKit for iPhone).

Figure 4.2 is an example of a thought record filled out by Angela, the woman introduced in Chapter 2 who struggled with sleep disturbance. Although Angela quickly resumed the activities she typically found pleasurable and meaningful, she found that her mood continued to be low and felt almost as if there was a black cloud following her. Until she completed the thought record, she did not realize the manner in which her thoughts about the loss were affecting her mood. Later in the chapter, I say more about the ways in which Angela dealt with the thoughts that she identified.

What if I can't figure out what I'm thinking? Most people are not in the habit of noticing their thinking, so it is logical that it might be difficult when you first embark on this exercise. As was stated previously, it could be that your cognitions are not in verbal format, but that instead they are in pictorial format. To access these mental images, you might ask yourself, "Am I remembering something

FIGURE 4.2. Angela's Three-Column Thought Record

Situation	Thought	Emotion and intensity (0 = lowest intensity; 10 = highest intensity)
Driving by hospital	I was robbed of happiness.	Despair (10)
Replaying the loss over and over in my mind	I should have caught the warning signs sooner.	Sadness (10) Self-loathing (10)
Annual employee's picnic at work	I'll fall apart. I can't face everyone.	Trepidation (10)
Walking by children's clothing section at a department store	Something is wrong with me; I caused the loss.	Sadness (10)
Partner is sitting quietly and seems to be staring into space.	I've failed him.	Sadness (10) Disappointment (10)
Interaction with family friend	She pitied me.	Anger (7)

horrible from the loss or trauma?" and "Am I imagining awful consequences for the future?"

Another strategy that you could use is simply to take a guess at what might be running through your mind. I find that most of the time, when my clients take a guess, the thoughts that they identify are ones that are reasonable given the demands of the situation. Angela's thought record in Figure 4.2 lists some common thoughts that people who have experienced reproductive loss often have. Do any of these thoughts sound familiar? If they seem vaguely familiar but still not quite right, do they prompt you to think of related thoughts that might be more accurate?

As you read through this chapter, you might find it tempting to skip the three-column thought record altogether and jump ahead in the process to get relief from your distressing thoughts. However, in my experience, people need some practice in simply identifying the most relevant thoughts associated with their emotional distress. Skipping over this practice runs the risk that you will find yourself working with thoughts that are only peripherally related to the key source of your distress. My recommendation is that you spend at least a few days on the three-column thought record before moving on to the exercises described in the remainder of this chapter. As you do this, see whether you run into the obstacles that I describe in the remainder of this section and apply the tools to overcome them.

What if I can focus only on how I feel, not what I am thinking? It is not uncommon to be so consumed by your emotional distress that it is difficult to focus on anything else. Between that and the fact that you might not be used to identifying your thoughts, it makes sense that you might need some practice with this exercise.

I would encourage you to be sure that what you are labeling is actually a feeling and not a thought. In today's society, we often use language that confuses thoughts and feelings, such as "I feel like a failure or I feel worthless." Even though we label failure and worthless as feelings, in actuality, they are thoughts: You are *perceiving* yourself as being a failure or as being worthless. When you do that, it's easy to take those perceptions of failure, worthlessness, and so on as fact, rather than as ideas that can be critically evaluated. When you catch yourself labeling a thought as a feeling, ask yourself, "When I have that idea or perception, how does that make me feel emotionally?" Exhibit 4.1 displays common emotional states experienced by people who have recently gone through a reproductive

EXHIBIT 4.1. Common Emotional States			
Depressed	Sad	Anxious	Alarmed
Disappointed	Discouraged	Panicked	Nervous
Ashamed	Guilty	Scared	Worried
Repugnant	Despicable	Frightened	Shaky
Disgusting	Irritated	Restless	Pained
Enraged	Hostile	Tortured	Dejected
Angry	Annoyed	Heartbroken	Sorrowful
Bitter	Resentful	Anguished	Unhappy
Inflamed	Infuriated	Lonely	Mournful
Indignant	Despair	Dismayed	Grieved
Fearful	Terrified		

loss. If the feeling that you believe you are experiencing is not on this list, consider the possibility that it might actually be a cognition (i.e., thought, perception, interpretation, or judgment) that you can work with in thought modification.

What if there are too many thoughts to sort out? It is true that you might be experiencing several thoughts, all of which are associated with different types of emotional distress. If you need to do so, please take several lines on the thought record to record as many as you believe are necessary.

One tip is to ask yourself, "What is the fundamental issue that is associated with my emotional distress?" or "What is the bottom line here?" It is often the case that the thoughts that you identify can be linked with an underlying theme or belief. Take a look at Angela's thoughts in Figure 4.2: "I was robbed of happiness, I can't face everyone, I caused the loss," and so on. When Angela asked herself what fundamental meaning might underlie this cluster of thoughts, she identified, "My life is tragic." She realized that this idea—that her life is tragic—was rearing its ugly head over and over in an array of specific situations. She now had words to put to the black cloud that she believed was following her.

Evaluating Distressing Thoughts and Images

As I stated earlier, the goal of thought modification is not simply to think positively. You don't need me to tell you that there is not a lot of positive associated with reproductive loss. However, it is important for you to critically evaluate the thoughts that you identify and examine the evidence that supports and refutes them so that you are not forgetting other factors that might soften the edges of your thinking, even just a little bit. If, after this critical evaluation, you determine that there are aspects of your thinking that are inaccurate, exaggerated, or otherwise unhelpful, then you can respond to them by constructing what therapists call a *balanced response*, or a new, adaptive thought that acknowledges what is unquestionably distressing as well as what might counteract some of the distress. After completing this exercise, you will still be grieving, and you will not be back to yourself. But it is my hope that the intensity of your emotional distress will have decreased a bit, which increases the likelihood that you will make decisions that will help you to take care of yourself and engage in pleasurable and valued activities.

You might start by asking yourself whether you are falling into one of the traps described earlier in the chapter. An affirmative response can serve as a red flag for you to slow down and take a look at your thinking before letting it spiral. In addition, you can ask many other questions that will help you evaluate the accuracy and helpfulness of the thoughts. The following are some questions you can ask yourself to get some distance from your thoughts and begin to evaluate them.

What evidence supports this thought? What evidence refutes this thought? When people examine the evidence that both supports and refutes their unhelpful thoughts, they are often forced to acknowledge that there is more evidence that refutes the thought than there is evidence that supports it. Angela applied this reasoning to get distance and perspective on her thought, "I was robbed of happiness." The evidence that supports that thought was, of course, that she experienced a painful loss. However, she also began to acknowledge many instances in her life in which she was rewarded with great happiness, such as graduating from college, finding someone whom she viewed as the perfect mate, and having several close-knit circles of friends from different times in her life. By examining the evidence, Angela realized that she was acknowledging only one component of happiness and that she was failing to recognize many sources of happiness that still existed in her life. Although her reproductive loss was indeed tragic, she acknowledged that her life, overall, was not.

Figure 4.3 is a worksheet called an *Evidence Log* that allows you to list the evidence associated with your unhelpful thoughts. You can jot down the emotionally distressing thought, the evidence that supports it, the evidence that refutes it, and the conclusion you draw on the basis of your examination of the evidence. Notice in the supportive evidence column that there is a caveat—"with reframe when necessary." This caveat was inserted because there are many instances in which people identify evidence that they believe supports their emotionally distressing thought, only to find that the evidence is not factual.

To illustrate this point, consider an instance in which Angela shared the news of her pregnancy loss with a family friend, and the family friend's response was to say how sorry she was and give Angela a hug. Later, Angela began to maintain an ongoing evidence log to evaluate the idea that people will pity her when they learn about the loss. She listed this experience with the family friend as evidence

FIGURE 4.3. Evidence Log

Thought	Evidence That Supports My Thought (with reframe when necessary)	Evidence That Refutes My Thought	Conclusion

that supported her prediction. A few weeks later, she shared her concerns with her mother and referenced this interaction with the family friend. Angela's mother was surprised at Angela's interpretation. The truth was that the family friend had also experienced a reproductive loss when she was younger, and Angela's news brought her back to that time. A more accurate interpretation of the family friend's behavior was that she was expressing empathy toward Angela, not that she had pitied her. This instance served as an important reminder that there might be other explanations that can account for the "evidence" that supports negative predictions. It also helped Angela to subsequently reach out to this family friend to obtain support from someone who was uniquely qualified to appreciate the pain that she was enduring.

What are other explanations? The previous discussion about Angela's evidence log illustrates just how easy it is to focus on one explanation for an event, forgetting about other explanations that are equally or even more likely. An *attribution* is the explanation we make for why an event happens. People who have experienced a reproductive loss often make attributions for their loss or trauma similar to those made by people who are depressed, such that their attributions are internal, global, and stable in nature.

Consider another entry on Angela's thought record—her reaction when she walked through the children's clothing section in the store, and she immediately said to herself, "I caused the loss. There is something wrong with me." This is an example of an internal attribution because she is attributing the sole cause of the loss to something being wrong with her, rather than to possible external factors, such as a random infection. When she begins this line of thinking, she often then says to herself, "Nothing ever goes the way I want it to go." This is an example of a global attribution because she is overgeneralizing to her entire life, rather than limiting her disappointment to the specific, isolated event that she experienced. Angela also says to herself, "This will never change," which is an example of a stable attribution because she regards her reproductive difficulties as an issue that will persist in the future, rather than as a temporary setback. Not surprisingly, when Angela makes internal, global, and stable attributions for upsetting life events, she experiences a great deal of emotional upset.

The opposite of internal, global, and stable attributions are those that are external, specific, and temporary in nature. For example, someone who experiences a pregnancy loss might attribute the loss to bad luck, rather than to herself (i.e., an external attribution); she might regard the loss as one specific disappointment, remaining mindful of the fact that other areas of her life are indeed going quite well (i.e., a specific attribution); and she might acknowledge the fact that many pregnancy losses are isolated incidents and that many women go on to have one or more healthy children (i.e., a transient attribution). These types of attributions are associated with less depression than internal, global, and stable attributions for negative life events. When you find yourself making internal, global, or stable attributions, be sure to ask yourself whether they have their basis in fact, such as information provided to your by your doctor, or whether you believe them because of how you are feeling (i.e., the emotional reasoning trap).

I often tell my clients that events we experience in our lives almost always have multiple causes. Rarely is there a single cause for an event. However, when we're struggling to find an explanation for events that are upsetting and that we don't understand, we often fall into the trap of making an overly simplistic attribution. Thus, I encourage my clients to ask the question, "What are other explanations for this event?" to begin to distance themselves from attributions that have the potential to be incorrect (e.g., internal attributions) and that perpetuate emotional distress. If it is still hard to attribute the event to anything other than internal, global, and stable causes, it might be helpful to run the explanations by a trusted family member or friend and see if he or she agrees with you.

What are the advantages of this way of thinking? the disadvantages? So far, we have considered instances in which one's thinking is overly focused on the negatives that perpetuate emotional distress at the expense of thinking that is focused on the positives, or at least the neutrals, that might balance out the negatives.

However, there are other instances in which people who have experienced reproductive loss find themselves ruminating on thoughts that are, indeed, quite accurate.

Consider Jill, who had gone through four cycles of intrauterine injections (IUI) with oral medications, one cycle of IUI with injectable medications, and four rounds of in vitro fertilization (IVF), all without conceiving. Two of the IVF rounds were covered by her insurance, and she and her husband paid for two out of pocket. She had few financial reserves for another round of IVF, and her doctor had gently informed her that the likelihood of another round being successful was low in light of the first four unsuccessful rounds.

It had been very important to Jill to have a child with her own egg rather than with a donor egg, and she was facing the possibility that this dream would not be realized. Understandably, she was extremely discouraged, and she found herself ruminating over the thought, "I'm never going to have a child with my own egg." Unfortunately, as time went on, the likelihood of this statement being true was higher and higher. It made sense that Jill was at a place in which she was faced with grieving the loss of the reproductive story that she had created, in which her child would be biologically related to her.

However, focusing on this fact kept Jill entrenched in her emotional distress and prevented her from broadening her mind to consider other options. Jill admitted that focusing on this thought usually just made her want to curl up in a ball and go back to bed. She isolated herself from others, skipping events with her extended family and even taking off some "mental health" days from work. Moreover, it moved her away from addressing the issues of having children rather than toward finding an alternative solution using the problem-solving skills that are described later in this book (see Chapter 8). Once Jill listed the specific ways in which ruminating on her thoughts made her situation worse, she was able to remember these ways each time she started going down that road, which motivated her to engage in some of the healthy behaviors described in previous chapters and some of the cognitive strategies described in this chapter.

The clarity of mind that she obtained from implementing these cognitive and behavioral strategies was that she was able to clarify her values (i.e., whether having a biologically related child was more important than having a child at all) and evaluate the advantages and disadvantages of alternative pathways (e.g., using a donor egg, using a surrogate, adopting, remaining without a child). She began to conclude that having a child who was not biologically related to her was not as catastrophic as she had assumed it would be when she first started her infertility treatments.

What would I tell a friend in this situation? Sometimes it is hard to distance ourselves emotionally from our thoughts. They feel so powerful, all consuming, and undeniably true that they overtake us. In these cases, it can be helpful for you to create distance by asking yourself what you would tell a friend in this situation. Asking this question can make your circumstances feel a little less personal.

One thing to watch out for, however, is the "yeah, buts" associated with negative comparisons to your friend. It is easy to fall into the trap of saying something like, "Yeah, but her situation is less dire than mine because. . . ." In my experience, the vast majority of the "yeah, buts" are our own interpretations of the implications of the differences between us and our friend rather than true facts. I find that the exercise of asking what we would tell a friend in this situation illustrates that we hold ourselves to very different standards than we do our friends and that there is no reason the standards can't be aligned.

If I must be in this awful situation, what meaning can I take away? What wisdom can I gain? How can I grow as a person? The derivation of meaning, wisdom, and personal growth from an experience like a reproductive loss can occur through many means. Perhaps it was the kindhearted nurse in the hospital who reminded you of the goodness of human nature. Perhaps it was the heartfelt sentiments sent by coworkers to whom, before this incident, you did not feel especially close. Perhaps it was the neighbor who reached out to you and disclosed that she, too, had experienced a horrific pregnancy loss. At times, the meaning that comes out of events like reproductive loss is the realization that people genuinely care.

In other instances, meaning, wisdom, and personal growth comes from the opportunity to weather adversity with grace and dignity. People who have experienced reproductive loss can make the choice to remain engaged with life, develop and cultivate passions, show gratitude toward their many blessings, and savor pleasant experiences. There will be many moments in which this seems impossible, and there will be many moments in which you just can't bring yourself to do this. No one is expecting you to be perfect. However, you can achieve great personal growth by learning how to handle tragedy in an adaptive manner. The truth is that you will likely experience some other type of loss or disappointment at some point in your life, and this experience, as awful as it is, can give you practice in learning to manage the emotional and psychological fallout.

Finally, meaning, wisdom, and personal growth can come from becoming involved in a cause that holds great meaning to you. I have met many women through my professional work who have started foundations to help survivors of pregnancy loss, preterm birth, and similar issues to help others who have gone through experiences that were similar to their own. Of course, you don't need to start a foundation to gain some meaning from your experiences. Perhaps you volunteer with an existing foundation. If that's too difficult for you, perhaps you can donate money to an existing foundation. Or you may volunteer your time or donate money (or both) to a foundation or nonprofit group that works with others who have experienced a different type of adversity in their lives (e.g., poverty, homelessness). The key here is that you attain greater meaning by being a part of a cause that is greater than yourself.

Developing a Balanced Response

The goal of thought modification is to ultimately develop a more balanced and helpful way of viewing your circumstances so that you will feel better. Consider the answers to the questions that were posed in the previous sections. If your responses suggest that there is a more balanced and helpful way of viewing your circumstances, then I invite you to develop a balanced response. A balanced response is the new perspective that takes into account the answers to one or more of these questions. Unlike the original thoughts, which are usually simple, specific, and direct (e.g., "This isn't fair"), the balanced response often contains several statements that represent a combination of answers to the evaluation questions that you contemplated. The complexity of the balanced response represents the complexity of the many nuances of the loss or trauma that you experienced. Balanced responses need to be compelling and believable, or they will be easy to simply dismiss. Responses such as "Just move on or Everything will be OK" usually won't help you to feel better because they do not acknowledge the pain you experienced or the uncertainty that you face.

How does one construct a balanced response? You simply piece together answers to the questions that you posed to evaluate the original thought. For example, if you used the evidence log in Figure 4.3, the conclusion that you drew at the close of the exercise might serve as the balanced response. Or the balanced response might include a combination of, say, the evidence that is inconsistent with the original thought, other explanations, and an acknowledgment of the wisdom you gain from being in this painful situation. Every balanced response is uniquely constructed on the basis of the answers to the evaluation questions that you found most helpful in creating distance from the original thoughts that were associated with so much emotional upset.

You can record balanced responses on a different version of the thought record called the *five-column thought record*. Figure 4.4

FIGURE 4.4. Five-Column Thought Record

Situation	Thought	Emotion and Intensity (0 = lowest intensity; 10 = highest intensity)	Balanced Response	New Emotion and Intensity (0 = lowest intensity; 10 = highest intensity)

is a blank five-column thought record for you to practice on, and Figure 4.5 is an example of Angela's completed five-column thought record. Like the three-column thought record, the five-column thought record allows room for you to record situations in which you experience emotional upset, the thoughts that ran through your mind, and the intensity of the specific emotions that you experienced. However, it contains an additional two columns. One of the new columns allows you to record the balanced response you arrived at as a result of the critical evaluation of the thought. In addition, it allows you to rerate your emotional intensity so that you have evidence that this process is indeed effective in managing your mood.

PROCESSING INTRUSIVE IMAGES OF THE LOSS

Some women experience pregnancy losses as traumatic events and continue to experience reminders of the event through intrusive memories, flashbacks, or nightmares, which cause the person to reexperience the trauma over and over. These reminders are usually experienced as horrific and terribly distressing. When people reexperience traumas in this way, they often attach a great deal of significance to these symptoms, which makes them feel even worse (e.g., "This means that I'm going crazy"). The significance attached to reexperiencing symptoms can be addressed using the thought modification techniques described in this chapter. For example, if a person believes that reexperiencing symptoms signifies that she is going crazy, a balanced response could be something like, "I went through a horrible experience that would be difficult for almost anyone to handle. These experiences are logical in light of what happened."

Actual intrusive memories, flashbacks, and nightmares can be handled in a different way if they continue to persist and cause emotional distress. According to trauma experts Barbara Rothbaum, Edna Foa, and Elizabeth Hembree, intrusive images persist because they are

FIGURE 4.5. Angela's Five-Column Thought Record

Situation	Thought	Emotional Intensity (0 = lowest intensity; 10 = highest intensity)	Balanced Response	New Emotion and Intensity (0 = lowest intensity; 10 = highest intensity)
Driving by hospital	I was robbed of happiness.	Despair (10)	My trauma will always be a part of my life that will make me sad when I focus on it. However, I have not fully been robbed of happiness, as I still get moments of joy when I am with my husband and my friends.	Despair (3) Optimism (2)
Replaying the loss over and over in my mind	I should have caught the warning signs sooner.	Sadness (10) Self-loathing (10)	My doctor told me many times that there is nothing I could have done to prevent this. Nobody blames me for the loss, and people have shown nothing but care and concern.	Sadness (7) Self-loathing (0)
Annual employee's picnic at work	I'll fall apart. I can't face everyone.	Trepidation (10)	I went to the picnic 2 years ago after my mother died and was worried about the same thing. There was so much going on that I did not even have time to think about her death.	No trepidation

Walking by children's clothing section at a department store	Something is wrong with me; I caused the loss.	Sadness (10)	The doctor said I did nothing wrong in the pregnancy. I must remember that a large percentage of women go through what I went through.	Sadness (4)
Partner is sitting quietly and seems to be staring into space	I've failed him.	Sadness (10) Disappointment (10)	The loss was not my fault. When I tell him that I think I have failed him, he always tells me this is not true.	Sadness (7) Disappointment (2)
Interaction with family friend	She pitied me.	Anger (7)	There could be a lot of other reasons why she hugged me. Maybe my loss struck a chord with her.	Anger (1)

incompletely processed—almost as if one opens a book to a random page but quickly decides that she doesn't like the book and shuts it. This is a form of avoidance that, unfortunately, allows the thoughts and feelings about the trauma to hang over a person like a black cloud in a threatening, menacing manner. The way to work through this cycle is to revisit the image, this time allowing detailed memories of the loss, without avoidance and in a safe environment, so that you learn that memories are painful and unpleasant but not dangerous. This process allows you to have more of a sense of control over the memories, rather than being in a position in which the memories control you. The technical term for this process is *imaginal exposure.*

In Chapter 7, I say more about the theory underlying exposure and the manner in which it helps people overcome avoidance. Although this process might sound daunting, there is a great deal of research evidence that supports its effectiveness. If you have persistent reexperiencing symptoms of your loss and experience these images as intrusive and disturbing, consider seeking the services of a cognitive behavioral therapist who can work with you to use imaginal exposure to help you process these images and memories.

WHY THIS WORKS

Thoughts are tricky. They are not fact; they are simply mental events that occur as a result of your neuronal activity. However, they can *feel* real, and they can be all consuming. The techniques described in this chapter work by making sure that you are viewing your life circumstances as factually, accurately, and helpfully as possible; in other words, it helps you to think about your life circumstances with balance. Again, there is no question that your reproductive loss was horrible—quite possibly, the most horrible experience you've gone through in your life. It would be ludicrous to ask you to "make lemonade out of lemons."

However, in my experience, when people are fixated exclusively on the terrible aspects of their loss or trauma, they forget about other aspects of their life that are meaningful and fulfilling. They forget to acknowledge the small encouraging aspects, such as the kindness of others. They don't see that their memories, while painful, are not dangerous. When I have my clients rate the degree of the intensity of their negative emotions associated with their negative thoughts on a 0-to-10 scale (0 = *low intensity*, 10 = *highest intensity possible*), not surprisingly, they usually give me a rating of 10. I find that when people rerate the intensity of their negative emotion after they consider their thoughts with as much balance as possible, the intensity drops a few points to, say, a 6 or a 7. No one is saying that a 6 or a 7 feels good—it doesn't. However, I find that it is much easier to begin to take care of oneself and engage in pleasurable or meaningful activities when one is at a 6 or a 7, rather than when at a 10. Moreover, thought modification has the potential to shift your focus of attention away from fixation or rumination on what happened and toward the present moment, allowing you to savor moments of pleasure and solve problems. In Chapter 9, I provide additional suggestions for ways to focus on the present rather than on the past.

CHAPTER 5

COPING WITH DISTURBING THOUGHTS AND IMAGES ABOUT THE FUTURE

In the previous chapter, we discussed ways of dealing with disturbing thoughts and images about the loss or trauma event itself and the immediate aftermath. In this chapter, we focus on ways of dealing with disturbing thoughts and images about the future—especially thoughts and images pertaining to future pregnancies, losses, unsuccessful attempts at fertility treatment or adoption, or life without a child. On the one hand, many people who have experienced reproductive loss find that the intensity of the thoughts and images about the loss or trauma event decreases with time. On the other hand, they may be facing decisions pertaining to childbearing, infertility, or adoption for many years to come, and the uncertainty of it all can be unbearable. Here I describe the manner in which the thought modification strategies described in the previous chapter can address these thoughts and images about the future. I also give you some suggestions for ways in which you can learn to tolerate, accept, and even embrace uncertainty.

COMMON TRAPS

As when thinking about the previous loss or trauma, people who have lost a child or who have undergone unsuccessful fertility treatments also can fall into traps when they face an uncertain future. This section describes these traps in detail.

Fortune-Telling

Fortune-telling is the tendency to predict the future. In many instances, anticipating the future is helpful and adaptive when making life decisions. For example, you need to plan ahead to save money to buy your first house, you need to plan ahead to get the schooling or training to enter into the profession of your choice, and so on. However, fortune-telling becomes a trap when you become convinced that a negative outcome will occur, and you take it as fact even though in the moment it is a hypothetical prediction. In these cases, it is easy to start feeling certain emotions (many of which are intense and distressing) and making decisions on the basis of this prediction even though there is no way to tell whether it will come true. The end result of fortune-telling is that you invest a great deal of mental energy ruminating over a negative outcome when, in many cases, it will never come to fruition. You also might end up making decisions that create a *self-fulfilling prophesy*, such that you take a course of action on the basis of expecting the negative outcome that increases the likelihood that the negative outcome will actually occur. People who fall prey to the fortune telling trap believe that they are guaranteed to experience the worst-case outcome, when in reality, the worst-case outcome occurs in only a tiny percentage of cases.

Consider Karen, who went through four unsuccessful trials of intrauterine insemination (IUI). She was convinced that other fertility treatments (e.g., in vitro fertilization [IVF]) would not work for her because of these failures. She proceeded with IVF, and the process was excruciating for her because she convinced herself that they would be unsuccessful. Thus, she went through many, many grueling months, which took a toll on her partner relationship.

Catastrophizing

Catastrophizing is the tendency to exaggerate the importance of something, such that it is viewed as a catastrophe or a disaster. I realize that most readers might be thinking, "but it IS a catastrophe if I don't have a child"—I know, because I had the same sorts of thoughts myself. I don't want to minimize the fact that it would feel devastating not to have a child if you desperately want one. However, in my experience, one of two things can happen when you start to go down this road. The first is something I call the *runaway train effect*—you begin imagining more and more awful consequences of the worst-case scenario of not having a child. Karen, for example, jumped from worry about not having a child to imagining herself alone on holidays, and then to being in a nursing home where every single resident except her had visits from children, grandchildren, and great-grandchildren. Thus, she catastrophized by running through images of her life that were likely very distorted, concluding that her entire life would be horrible and that she would be all alone because she didn't have a child.

All-or-Nothing Thinking

All-or-nothing thinking is the tendency to think in extremes or poles, like black and white rather than shades of gray. All-or-nothing thinking causes trouble for us because it is an inaccurate representation of the world—rarely is anything that we experience all good or bad and not the other. Moreover, many people who engage in all-or-nothing thinking tend to veer toward the negative end of the pole, concluding that they are a failure, that things will never get better, or that life is meaningless. Those are powerful self-statements that are sure to be associated with emotional upset in almost anyone. When you catch yourself using words such as *always* or *never*, consider the possibility that you are falling into the all-or-nothing thinking trap. Karen's catastrophic images of the future also reflected all-or-nothing thinking, as she concluded that she would be alone and that her life would be totally devoid of joy without having a child. Although it was true that there was a possibility that she would not be a mother, her conclusion that she would be "alone" negated the important roles that her partner and her close friends played in her life.

Overgeneralization

Overgeneralization is the tendency to see a single negative event as a never-ending pattern. Many, many women who have miscarriages or neonatal losses are convinced that they will have miscarriages or neonatal losses with each subsequent pregnancy. It is not difficult to see why she would fall into this pattern of thinking, and in reality, a previous reproductive loss does put most women at higher risk than average for another reproductive loss. However, most women who have miscarriages go on to have successful pregnancies. In fact, when I did my own research on the probability of a pregnancy loss after miscarriage or neonatal death, I was shocked to learn that most women who have *multiple* losses still go on to have successful pregnancies. Thus, as hard as it is, it is important to take the loss or trauma as a single negative event unless you have medical evidence to support the notion that this will be an ongoing problem for you.

I also hear instances of overgeneralizing when people conclude that because they experienced a pregnancy loss or reproductive trauma, it means that *many* things in their lives will also not work out for them. Here, it is important to remember that difficulties in one aspect of a person's life do not have to be equivalent to difficulties in multiple aspects of one's life. This is another example that illustrates that it is easy to zero in on the negative and forget about the neutrals and positives in one's life.

"Should" Statements

Should statements can rear their ugly heads when you are thinking about the future as well as when you are thinking about the past loss or trauma. In many instances, they manifest when people think of what their lives "should" look like (e.g., two children and a house with a white picket fence). As I stated in the previous chapter, *should* statements are problematic because they fail to account for life's unexpected events and challenges. Because they are inflexible, one's response to stressors that interfere with the *should* statements is to be angry, disappointed, and anxious. They keep you from achieving acceptance of your situation as it is. I highly encourage you to have several visions for the way you'd like your life to turn out, accounting for various obstacles and emphasizing the positives in each scenario.

Positive Beliefs About Worry

Recent research by Concordia University professor Michel Dugas and his colleagues suggests that one reason people worry and ruminate about the future is because they believe that doing so is beneficial. For example, some people believe that worrying about the future helps them to find solutions to their problems. However, in actuality, worrying about the future has the potential to create enough anxiety to interfere with problem solving because it is difficult to think clearly and systematically and to see all possibilities that could serve as solutions to problems. Moreover, worry is not a cognitive process that proceeds in a linear manner that leads to a solution to one's problems. Instead, it recycles over and over in one's mind, such that one rehashes over and over the implications of future catastrophes.

Other people believe that by worrying, they are preparing themselves for the worst and somehow buffering themselves from negative emotions. It is almost as if they believe that they "invest" themselves in negative emotions now, they will have to "pay" less when the worst-case scenario actually occurs. It is true that worrying allows for people not to build false or overstated expectations for an unsuccessful outcome. However, what this argument ignores is that during the time in which a person is worrying about the future, she is experiencing a great deal of negative emotion. Thus, worry doesn't serve as a buffer at all; in fact, it creates excessive negative emotion. It also takes people away from appreciating and savoring the present moment because they are wrapped up "in their heads."

I have also heard people say that worrying about the future actually prevents bad things from happening; "after all, every other time in my life that I've worried, nothing bad has happened, so I'm not going to mess with my track record this time." The problem with this argument is that it does not account for the fact that bad things happen only a small percentage of the time, and it is likely a worst-case scenario would not have occurred even in the absence of worry. Thus, people who carry this belief are subjecting themselves to an untestable hypothesis because they do not learn that there is no relation between worry and the absence of worst-case scenarios.

People who have experienced reproductive loss with whom I have worked often understand, in theory, that these are false beliefs. However, I also commonly hear that in the case of childbearing, the stakes are too high not to be worried. It is understandable that concerns, worries, and fears about childbearing might persist for several years until there is a resolution (i.e., you have a child, you have multiple children, or you don't have a child). However, a key to taking care of yourself during this uncertain time is to approach these worries with balance and ensure that they are not so consuming that they prevent you from living your life and obtaining a sense of pleasure, accomplishment, and meaning from your activities.

STEPS TO THOUGHT MODIFICATION

The steps for modifying disturbing thoughts and images about an uncertain future are quite similar to the steps for modifying disturbing thoughts or images about the loss or trauma event and its aftermath. First, you identify the disturbing thoughts and images, perhaps using a tool like the three-column thought record. Figure 5.1 displays

FIGURE 5.1. Karen's Three-Column Thought Record

Situation	Thought	Emotion (0 = lowest intensity; 10 = highest intensity)
Learning about rates of successful IVF	IVF will be unsuccessful.	Anxiety (10) Despair (10)
Thinking about the possibility of failed IVF.	I'll end up all alone.	Fear (10)
Noticing the children at the neighborhood barbeque	I'll be the only woman in the neighborhood who does not have a child.	Anxiety (10) Depression (10)
Partner is spending the evening on the computer in the other room	I'm driving her away by being so obsessed with all of this. I'll lose her.	Despair (10)

a three-column thought record that Karen completed. Notice that, without fail, she rated the intensity of her emotional experiences as a 10 out of 10. This is not uncommon when worrying about an uncertain future.

Second, you evaluate the thoughts, and if necessary, modify them to be more balanced, accurate, or helpful. Questions that you can begin to ask yourself are as follows:

What's the worst that can happen? the best? the most realistic? It is easy to get caught up in the worst-case outcome when worrying about an uncertain future. When this occurs, it's important to spend an equal amount of time considering the best-case outcome, as well as the most realistic outcome. In most instances when I have done this myself or coached my clients in responding truthfully to these questions, they find that the most realistic outcome is much closer to the best-case outcome than the worst-case outcome. Moreover, they also realize that the most realistic outcome is one that is generally good or one they could readily accept.

Jill, introduced in the previous chapter, asked herself these questions when her fertility doctor advised against additional trials of IVF using her own egg. Her worst-case outcome was that she would not have a child, and her best-case outcome was that she would overcome the odds, get pregnant on her own, and carry the child to term. However, given her history of unsuccessful fertility treatments, the most realistic outcome was that she would have to use a donor egg or consider adoption. Although Jill was disappointed that the most realistic outcome involved the fact that she would not be biologically related to her child, she eventually decided that it was most important to her to have a child by any means necessary. She also recognized that plenty of people have children through donor eggs or choose to adopt and that these people have healthy relationships with their children and that there are many resources available for sharing this news with their children.

What is the likelihood of the worst-case scenario? When we worry about the future, we tend to overestimate the probability of bad things happening to us. I recently worked with a client who was petrified that a gunman would enter her child's preschool and that her son would be a casualty. Her anxiety was severe enough that she began to keep him home with school despite his protests that he wanted to go to school and see his friends. She did some research and calculated the probability of this happening by estimating the number of children who attend school in the state of Pennsylvania, as well as the number of school shootings that had occurred in the state. Her calculation led her to conclude that there was approximately a 1 in 250 million chance that her son would be killed in a school-shooting incident. She then coupled this statistic with the fact that her son did not attend preschool on a full-time basis and estimated that, given the time he was actually in school, he had a 1 in 800 million chance that he would be killed in a school shooting incident. Although one can never rule out the possibility of a tragedy like this happening, my client realized that the odds were low enough that she was causing more damage by preventing her son from engaging in an activity that was appropriate for his social and emotional development.

The odds are not so small for pregnancy loss and reproductive traumas. Nevertheless, as I stated earlier in this chapter, my own research led me to see that many, many women go on to have successful pregnancies even if they had more than one devastating loss. It just doesn't feel like that but this possibility may well seem remote after such a loss (i.e., emotional reasoning). Conversely, it is generally the case that odds are much less than 50% that any single fertility treatment will be successful (unless a donor egg is used). Those odds can be disheartening for many people. Nevertheless, the odds of a single fertility treatment being successful are usually greater than the odds of getting pregnant without the fertility treatment, a fact that is important to keep in mind. If it is helpful for you to think about the odds or the likelihood, as it was for my client, then by all means use this strategy. However, if you don't think it would be helpful to calculate the odds or likelihood (or if you do so over, and over, and over in your mind), keep reading. It may be that some other approaches to evaluating the likelihood and impact of a worst-case scenario occurring will be a better match for you. It also might be the case that reflecting on a combination of these questions will be the most thorough approach to addressing your worries about an uncertain future.

How bad would the worst-case outcome actually be? This might seem like a strange question to ask because pregnancy losses and infertility would be regarded as very bad by almost anyone. However, this question might be appropriate to ponder in some cases. For example, for as long as she could remember, Amelia had a vision of having a rather large family with at least four children. Now, she was struggling to have one, and she was facing the possibility that she would not have the family of which she had dreamed. Although it took some time for her to come to terms with the loss of this dream, she realized that there were many advantages of having a small family with, say, one child. For example, she began to consider the financial implications of having a smaller family, and she realized that some advantages of having one child were that she and her husband would be able to pay his or her college tuition in full and save enough for retirement that their child would not need to worry about taking care of them when they got older. Thus, there is no question that you would have to manage the grief associated with a worst-case outcome if it were to occur, but there might be some unexpected positives that you are overlooking.

How would I cope if the worst-case outcome were to occur? This question is an important one. Many people who fear a worst-case outcome have the general sense that they would fall apart or that their lives would be empty, failing to envision the specific manner in which they would cope. It's no wonder, then, that the worst-case outcome is so threatening. Thus, I encourage you to have a *decatastrophizing plan* (similar to the decatastrophizing statement described in Chapter 2) that lays out, specifically, what you will do to cope if the worst-case outcome were to occur. Many people find that having a decatastrophizing plan gives them the sense of controllability and predictability that they're so desperately searching for. It helps them to see that although a worst-case outcome is far from desired, they can survive it and make the most of the circumstances that they have been dealt.

Figure 5.2 presents Amelia's decatastrophizing plan, which summarizes the specific manner in which she would raise her child as well as things to be mindful of in the event that she is able to have only one child. Amelia felt a great deal of relief after constructing her decatastrophizing plan. She realized that if she were to have only one child, although life would be very different from what she had envisioned, it would not be the end of the world, and there were

---

FIGURE 5.2. Amelia's Decatastrophizing Plan

Amelia's Decatastrophizing Plan

- Take some time to grieve the loss of my dream of having many children.
- Make a great effort to spend time with other families in the neighborhood and at my child's school.
- Make a great effort to have my child develop a special relationship with his or her cousins across the country.
- Implement special family traditions that the three of us can enjoy and look forward to.
- Take the time to express gratitude for the child I do have.
- Invest money wisely in the child's college plan and in our retirement.
- Be mindful of the advantages of having one child (e.g., finances, we'll be able to fully be there for our child in all of his or her activities).

several ways in which she could ensure that the family unit was a close and supportive one and that her child would develop meaningful relationships with others.

If you are worried about not having even one child, then you can create a different type of decatastrophizing plan. Describe all of the valued activities that you would pursue in the event that you don't have children. Create a vision of a life filled with passions, meaning, and close relationships.

Does _____ have to lead to or equal to _____? This question is terrific for people who tend to believe that certain events carry profound (and usually negative) meaning or are destined to lead to an awful fate. Jill, for example, struggled with the idea that she was less of a woman because she was struggling with infertility. By asking herself if fertility struggles necessarily equaled being less of a woman, she saw that infertility said nothing about her personally and that she had plenty of characteristics that made her a successful, worthy person. Amelia, in contrast, worried that having an only child meant that the child would grow up to be spoiled, unskilled, and/or lonely. After doing some reading on the topic, however, she learned that the research does not bear this out, and she went back to her decatastrophizing plan to see that there are many things that she can do as a parent to avoid these unfavorable outcomes.

What's the effect of believing my automatic thought? What's the effect of changing my thinking? Letting go of unhelpful negative thinking can be incredibly difficult when the stakes are so high. Many people report being consumed with thoughts about pregnancy, losses, and fertility treatment for months and even years until they finally have a child or have decided to stop trying. If this describes you, consider asking yourself the questions posed in this section— "What's the effect of believing my automatic thoughts? What's the effect of changing my thinking?" By critically examining your answers to these questions, you may see that the effect of your thinking, even if it is largely accurate, is to bring you down and take you away from living in the present moment. The effects of changing your thinking, or at least focusing on something other than the "what-ifs," could mean that you obtain some joy and pleasure in your life despite the awful loss or trauma that you experienced, that you reconnect with your partner, and that you find meaning in the pain that you experienced.

What should I do about it? In many ways, you're doing everything you can about your situation. When pregnant, you're eating healthfully, you're staying away from alcohol and drugs, you're avoiding certain foods that could cause an infection, and so on. If you're struggling with infertility, you're gathering information, perhaps consulting with a fertility specialist and going through diagnostic tests. In those instances, asking this question will not be helpful because you already are doing so much to address your situation.

On the other hand, you might be experiencing some distressing thoughts that you *can* do something about that you might not be recognizing. Karen, for example, worried that she was driving away her partner because she was so fixated on having a child. It would certainly be unsettling to worry about the threat of loss of the partner relationship in addition to dealing with the uncertainty of one's reproductive future. However, by asking herself what she should do about her strained relationship, Karen remembered that she and her partner had gone through difficult times in the past and that she had made some adjustments that ultimately repaired the relationship. For example, in the past, she took care to show interest in her partner's life—particularly how her partner was managing a stressful career, she arranged for a relaxing couple's spa weekend, and she suggested that they have a weekly "date night." Her partner had been quite receptive to these expressions of love, and their relationship quickly got back on track. Although Karen continued to experience a great deal of stress associated with uncertainty about her reproductive future, she concluded that there was no reason she could not implement similar things to nurture their relationship during this difficult time.

Developing Balanced Responses

Just as you saw in the previous chapter, what you're aiming to do with these evaluation questions is to use them in the service of developing a balanced response. Remember that the balanced response is not just positive thinking; positive thinking in the context of pregnancy loss or infertility is simply unrealistic. Rather, you will construct a balanced response on the basis of your responses to a combination of the evaluation questions, taking care to address all of the complexities of the circumstances that you are facing. The following are some of the balanced responses that Karen, Jill, and Amelia developed as they worked through these thought modification exercises:

- Karen: IVF will be unsuccessful (automatic thought). → In looking at the data given to me by the fertility clinic, there is a reasonable chance that IVF will work. In addition, my insurance covers two IVF cycles, so I know that I will get at least two tries. In the event that it is unsuccessful, we will consider adopting. There is no question that there is a long road ahead, but there is more than one way for us to have a child (balanced response).
- Karen: I'll be the only woman in the neighborhood who does not have a child (automatic thought). → This statement simply is not true, and I'm falling into the all-or-nothing thinking trap. The neighbor who lives across the street is in her 40s and does not have children. She and her husband are living a wonderful life by traveling and pursuing interests they are passionate about. Besides, I haven't even gone through IVF yet, so I'm fixating on something that hasn't even occurred yet (balanced response).

- Jill: It is a tragedy that I won't be biologically related to my child (automatic thought). → It's true that my dream was to have a child to whom I am biologically related. But the most important thing is that I have a child. I might still be able to carry the child even if I am not biologically related. Many women go through the same thing and have close, bonded relationships with their children (balanced response).
- Karen: I'm driving my partner away by being so obsessed with having a child (automatic thought). → It is true that there has been some tension in our relationship lately. However, during our commitment ceremony, we took the vow to stay with each other through thick and thin. We've had some tough times before, and we've always gotten through them. I know what adjustments I made before when we had tough times, and I can make the same adjustments now (balanced response).
- Amelia: Being an only child means that the child will be spoiled, unskilled, and lonely (automatic thought). → Research suggests that only children are no more spoiled, unskilled, or lonely than children who have siblings. In fact, I even read somewhere that only children are closer to their parents than children with siblings, and I would love to have a very close relationship with my child. There are many things I can do to ensure that my child has close relationships with others, such as fostering close relationships with families in the neighborhood and at his or her school (balanced response).

ACCEPTANCE OF UNCERTAINTY

Most people are uncomfortable with uncertainty, even uncertainty about small things, like going to a movie without knowing what it is about or reading any reviews. With childbearing, the uncertainty is amped up 100-fold. Many people regard having children as the single most important goal in their lives, and it can be unbearable not to know whether their dreams will come true. The problem that occurs when people have trouble accepting uncertainty is that they usually veer toward the negative implications of uncertainty—that the desired outcome will not occur, that they will experience a devastating loss or tragedy, that they will not be able to handle problems that are thrown their way, and so on. However, it is important to realize that uncertainty is not equivalent to bad things happening. The other side of the coin with uncertainty is that the doors have opened for good things to happen. Remaining open to the possibility that good things can happen has the potential to balance out the emotional distress associated with the prediction that uncertainty leads to negative outcomes.

It would behoove all of us to become more accepting of uncertainty because uncertainty is about the only thing in life that is actually guaranteed. One way to become more comfortable with uncertainty is to intentionally place yourself in the circumstances for which the outcome is uncertain. Go to the movie even though you know nothing about the plot and have not read reviews. Try a cuisine or a restaurant that is new to you. Take a new route home from work even though you do not know whether you will hit traffic. Spend a long weekend at a new location rather than going to the same beach or cabin in the mountains.

You might ask what these simple tasks have to do with the enormity of the uncertainty of your reproductive future. I'd have the same reaction. The overarching goal of these sorts of tasks is to become more comfortable with uncertainty: The more you place yourself in situations or circumstances that are uncertain, the less you will feel threatened by them. In addition, you may begin to gather evidence that there are many times when you are faced with uncertainty and that the outcome is surprisingly favorable. These experiences will help ease the alarm when you are faced with uncertainty about more substantial situations, such as your reproductive future.

WHY THIS WORKS

As I stated in the previous chapter, thought modification works because it helps people ensure that their thinking is as accurate, helpful, and balanced as is possible. When facing an uncertain reproductive future, thought modification can help you (a) confirm that you are thinking realistically about the odds of an unwelcome event occurring, (b) develop a decatastrophizing plan so that you know exactly how you would cope a worst-case outcome if it occurs, (c) recognize ways that you successfully overcame problems or dealt with uncertainty in the past and consider how you would apply them in the present moment, and (d) acknowledge the pieces of a worst-case outcome that could nevertheless contribute to a meaningful life.

It is so easy to become consumed with the what-ifs of an uncertain reproductive future. "What if I experience another loss? What if I don't have the number of children that I had always dreamed about? What if I can't have a biological child of my own? What if I end up not having children at all?" No one would blame you for ruminating over these and other what-ifs. However, ultimately what happens is that the fixation becomes the center of your life, taking you away from other sources of joy and meaning, such as your partner relationship, relationships with other family members and friends, your career, and your other passions. In other words, your struggle against the inherent uncertainty of your reproductive future is taking you away from your life in the present moment. Not only does that make you vulnerable to emotional distress like depression and anxiety, it can make future attempts at pregnancy and fertility treatment excruciating. My wish for you, if you must be reeling from such a tragic loss, is that you put yourself in a position to savor the moments of joy and pleasure that come your way that you very much deserve. You can only identify those moments if you are living in the present, rather than fixating on the what-ifs of the future. In Chapter 9, I say more about ways to live mindfully in the present to achieve this.

CHAPTER 6

INTERACTING WITH OTHERS

Interactions with others can be extremely daunting for people who have experienced a reproductive loss. Concerns you might be experiencing range from wondering how to share the news to others, to worrying that others will say something insensitive (which invariably happens), to worrying about how you will react to your friends and acquaintances who are pregnant or who have healthy children. You might feel like you want to avoid interactions with others forever. Eventually, though, you will be in a position in which you are going to resume usual activities in your life, such as going back to work, going shopping, and connecting with family and friends.

This chapter describes the common concerns you might have about interacting with others. I open this chapter with a section called "Communication 101," which describes an assertive communication style and contrasts it with other, less helpful communication styles. I refer to the assertive communication style as I describe ways to consider handling uncomfortable interactions with others. I also link back to the thought modification skills that you learned about in previous chapters because they might be of assistance as you implement assertive communication. Toward the end of the chapter, I examine the manner in which refraining from social isolation and utilizing social support have the potential to improve mood and promote healing. My hope is that after reading this chapter, you will have a more specific idea of how you will approach these interactions and more confidence in yourself in saying what's important to you to say. The first time interacting with people after a reproductive loss is never easy. But I'm hopeful that these strategies will help you to best take care of yourself and maintain your relationships with others.

COMMUNICATION 101

Much of what I present in this chapter are examples of an assertive communication style. *Assertiveness* means that you communicate in a manner that confidently acknowledges your needs and rights as well as the needs and rights of others. It is being true to yourself, your needs, and your opinions without trampling over or disregarding the needs and the rights of other people. In other words, assertive communication is balanced communication. Just as I advocated for balanced thinking in the previous two chapters, I also advocate for a balanced approach to communication. People who are assertive present themselves in a manner in which they appear confident, honest, and authentic. They approach interactions with the attitude "I have every right to state how I feel or what I need. And, at the same time, I respect others who may view the situation differently."

Assertive communication can be contrasted with passive, aggressive, and passive–aggressive approaches to communication. *Aggressive* communication occurs when a person advocates for her own needs and rights above all others, usually disregarding the perspectives and opinions of others. People who are aggressive often believe that their needs are more important than the needs of others or that their time is more valuable than that of others. People who adopt an aggressive communication style often appear arrogant or threatening to others.

Passive communication, in contrast, occurs when a person fails to advocate for her own needs and rights and allows others to make decisions for her, even decisions that pertain to her own well-being. Many people who adopt a passive communication style believe that they must do so to avoid conflict with other people, lest they might be rejected or abandoned by others. At times, people who adopt a passive communication style do so because they believe that by asserting themselves, they will hurt others' feelings, which would just make them feel guilty. Still others who adopt a passive communication style believe that they do not deserve to make requests of others or assert their own opinion.

Finally, a *passive–aggressive* communication style is one in which a person does not directly state her needs to others but instead engages in subtle behaviors to communicate her needs. Many people who adopt a passive aggressive communication style overtly say one thing to others but really mean something different and will go behind the scenes to get their needs met. Some regard people who present with a passive aggressive personality style as manipulative or "gamey." In my experience, many people who present in a passive aggressive manner are not intentionally trying to manipulate others; rather, they dislike confrontation, much like many people who adopt a passive communication style, but they also believe their needs should be met, much like a person who adopts an assertive communication style. In my mind, the key is to be as direct and aboveboard as possible with communication so that all parties have similar expectations for the interaction and interpretations of what is happening between them. This will be in your best interest at times when communication has the potential to be particularly difficult, such as when you are recovering from a reproductive loss.

Notice that many of the factors that underlie these communication styles are beliefs—beliefs about conflict with others, beliefs about the self, and so on. All of the beliefs can be evaluated using the thought modification strategies described in Chapters 4 and 5. It is often the case that orienting yourself using these thought modification strategies can help you to become centered so that you put your best foot forward as you attempt to communicate an important message to others. For example, if you have the belief that you need to take care of others who might be upset about the reproductive loss, you can use the thought modification strategies to adopt a more balanced view such as, "I have every right to take care of myself first during this devastating time, and I will encourage others to take care of themselves in their own ways as well."

The other important point to remember about communication is that it consists of overt verbal, subtle verbal, and nonverbal pieces. In other words, it's not just *what* you say that is important, but *how* you say it. When considering what you say (i.e., overt verbal communication), it can also be helpful to be cognizant of your tone of voice, the loudness of your voice, the speed at which you speak your words, and your voice inflection (i.e., subtle verbal communication). These factors can reinforce your message if they are consistent with what you are communicating. Conversely, they can diminish the impact of your message if they are inconsistent with what you are communicating. Consider, for example, the person who makes a request (e.g., "I'd like some time to myself") but then ends the request on a high pitch, as if she is asking a question. That pitch could very well communicate that she is asking permission from the other person for her request, rather than stating it outright.

I realize that you are likely not reading this book for a full-fledged lesson on communication and that now is not the time to perfect the fine art of communication. The reason I'm sharing these with you is so that your communications to and requests of others are made as effectively as possible, so that you have to repeat them as few times as is possible, and so that you maximize the likelihood that others will understand crystal clear what you are saying and asking and follow through with your request. This can be a time when it is tough to know exactly what you want to communicate, let alone how you might go about communicating, so it is my hope that this chapter will give you some tips.

CONCERNS ABOUT INTERACTING WITH OTHERS

Interacting with others following a reproductive loss brings many challenges. Of course, sharing news about the loss over and over means that you are being reminded of the loss over and over. In addition, you can't control the reactions of others. Because it is so difficult to understand the enormity of a reproductive loss, people do not have a socially accepted script to follow. What this means is that they might very well say something that just makes you feel worse. In fact, it might even be the case that someone responds to you with a great deal of empathy and sensitivity, and it *still* feels like that person said or did the wrong thing. For a time, it might feel like nothing others can say will be of comfort to you. In this section, I share some of the common scenarios reported by people who experienced reproductive loss.

Sharing the News With Others

Likely the first task you will face following a reproductive loss is sharing the news with other people. Many of these people might have been eagerly anticipating another addition to the family or circle of friends. It is understandable that this task is daunting; after all, you have to speak the words out loud. You have to manage your own emotional reaction as you speak the words out loud. And then, you likely might see there is a need to help others manage their own reactions to the news. Keeping all of these pieces in mind when you are at a low point can seem like too much.

FAMILY. Although many people view their family members as the people who give them the most unconditional support, sharing news about a reproductive loss with family members can be particularly challenging. Your parents and your partner's parents were probably looking forward to grandparenting the new child. Your siblings and your partner's siblings might have been looking forward to being an uncle or an aunt to the new child. In other words, they likely had their own reproductive stories that spoke to the roles that they had hoped to play in the new child's life. It is logical, therefore, that they will also experience a sense of loss.

If there is one thing I hope that you take away from this chapter, it is this: *You are not responsible for the reactions of others to the reproductive loss.* Too often, I hear that people feel so guilty that their loved ones are upset about the loss, they spend more time comforting them than taking care of themselves. They are allowed to grieve and experience emotional distress. However, right now, your first priority is taking care of yourself. It is their responsibility to figure out the best way to take care of themselves.

There is no easy way to put the news into actual words. Some people find that it is helpful to share the news with one trusted family member and then to have that family member inform others. Others find that they can handle sharing the news with their own family but that they would prefer their partner share the news with his or her family. Just know that you can choose whatever method of communication works for you.

You may want to surround yourself with your family members, or you may want to hold off on seeing them in person for a bit. Again, there is no right or wrong decision about this; only you know what you are ready for. If you'd like some time to yourself before having in-person contact with your family, you might consider saying something like, "I know how difficult this is for all of us as a family. And what I think would help me the most right now is to take a few days to myself so that I can digest everything that's happened. I will let you know when I am ready to start being around people." You might frame this request in a way that it comes across as a statement, rather than asking permission from others to confirm that this is OK with them. This is one example of assertive communication.

There are a few key elements of this example, which will be evident in many of the suggestions that I have peppered throughout this chapter. Take a look at the first sentence: "I know how difficult this is for all of us as a family." This is a statement that acknowledges and validates the pain that your family members are likely to be feeling. Often, people are more open to hearing what you have to say if they feel validated and understood. Now take a look at the second sentence: "And what I think would help me the most right now is for me to take a few days to myself so that I can digest everything that's happened." This is an example of an assertive statement that clearly defines what you are requesting. Notice that this statement is made in a definite but nonthreatening manner. It's not giving the message that you'd like the other family members to "back off!" It's simply stating what would be best for you. Finally, take a look at the third sentence: "I will let you know when I am ready to start being around people." This statement clarifies the parameters of next step—that you will take the lead in letting them know when you are ready for more contact.

When I work with my clients to develop an assertive communication style, they often agree, in theory, that the approach seems sound, but they question their ability to actually implement it. After all, many people have family dynamics characterized by heavily entrenched communication patterns and expected roles that family members follow. Your mother may be the caretaker. Your father may be the head of the household who believes he knows what's best. Your sister may be the "practical one." Your brother might be the "immature one." On the one hand, I realize that your view of these roles and corresponding interactional patterns developed on the basis of your very real past experiences. The communication style that I'm suggesting may be inconsistent with the communication style that has emerged from the role you play in your family. It may feel awkward to implement it now, during a crisis.

However, on the other hand, I would encourage you not to prejudge whether the communication strategies described in this chapter will be successful because you might draw a conclusion such as, "What's the use? They won't listen anyway." When you draw such a conclusion, you decrease the likelihood that you use assertive communication, and you increase the likelihood that you do not get your own unique needs met. Give your family members credit that they will step up to the plate and respect your assertive communication when it counts, such as in the time after a reproductive loss. And if they don't step up to the plate, know that you are still allowed to be assertive, communicate your needs, and set boundaries.

FRIENDS. In some ways, it might be easier to tell your close friends of the reproductive loss than it is to tell family. They might be the people to whom you have already told your deepest feelings, hopes, wishes, and dreams. They also might be a little bit less personally invested in your offspring than your family members. They might be able to help you engage in the pleasurable activities that I discussed in Chapter 2, and they could serve as a coach in achieving the balanced thinking that I described in Chapters 4 and 5.

In my experience, there are two sets of circumstances that have the potential to be problematic in interactions with friends. These circumstances do not necessarily arise immediately after sharing the news, but they might arise in the aftermath. First, it is possible that you will perceive the reactions of and support offered by some friends to be less than ideal. For example, perhaps a good friend calls you and offers support when she hears the news, but then you do not hear from her for several weeks. It is logical that you might feel hurt and wonder why she did not reach out to you more during this difficult time. You might even conclude that she is not as good of a friend as you thought she was.

Remember the thought modification question that I posed in Chapter 4—"Can there be any other explanations?" Before you decide to write off this friend, critically evaluate the answer to that question. Might this event have triggered a memory of something aversive that your friend experienced in her own life, such as the death of a family member? Is your friend going through an extraordinary amount of stress right now? Is your friend a bit socially awkward, such that she often doesn't know how to respond to difficult situations? In my experience, it proves to be the case that many friends just don't know what to say or what to do. They wonder whether they will make things worse, whether they'd be somehow bothering you, or whether they're overstepping the roles that family members should play. True, it would be nice if they reached out anyway, but at least the reason behind their lack of contact is not a lack of care or concern. Thus, giving your friend the benefit of the doubt can help reduce anger, disappointment, and hurt. Even if the friend in question has a history of dropping off the face of the earth when the going gets tough, don't worry about making a decision about the fate of the friendship right now. Just concentrate on connecting with the people who have reached out to you and who you can accept into your grieving process for the time being.

The second circumstance that can be problematic pertains to friends who are pregnant or who have one or more small children. It's easy to find yourself in a catch-22 situation in which you are truly happy for your friend but in which it is extraordinarily difficult to be around her because she is a constant reminder of what you don't have. What's more, you might have *several* friends who are at varying stages in their childbearing journeys, and it might seem as if it's going easily for all of them except for you. In these instances, you might be anticipating upcoming baby showers and wondering how in the world you will be able to get through them.

Almost anybody who is pregnant or who is a mother will understand your anguish. My bet is that if you need to distance yourself from one or more of these friends for the time being, they will understand. Here is another place where sensitive yet assertive communication would be in order. You might say something like, "I hope you know that you are a dear friend and your friendship means the world to me. And right now, reminders of children are just too much for me. Would it be OK with you if we take contact with one another at my own pace right now?" Look at the components of this piece of communication—first validation, then an explanation of what you are going through, and then a request for certain boundaries. By prefacing the request with validation and an explanation of where you are coming from, you are assuring your friend that you value the friendship and that less contact than usual should not be taken personally.

Of course, it will be important to reconnect with any friends from whom you distance yourself after a period of time. When you are a true friend, you recognize that others have needs, too. Friendship is about sharing experiences and providing support even when it is hard. The cognitive and behavioral strategies described in this book will help you to do so.

COLLEAGUES. Although most of us are not as close with our colleagues as we are with our friends, it can be extraordinarily difficult to share the news with colleagues (and sometimes clients) because, if you work outside of the home, they have born witness to your pregnancy from its early stages. Many women who have experienced a pregnancy loss report dread about going back into the office, when it is clear from their appearance that they are no longer pregnant. They imagine the faces full of pity, the hushed voices, the tiptoeing around. Moreover, there is a similar issue that you might face with friends who are pregnant—if you have colleagues who are pregnant or who have small children, then you will be continually reminded of your loss.

Sharing the news of the loss with colleagues has the potential to be a bit more straightforward than it is with friends and family. Many of you can probably e-mail one contact person, such as your supervisor or the office manager, and let that person take care of notifying others. Be prepared to get some offers of condolences—flowers, e-mail or voicemail messages, and the like. Although these gestures are heartfelt, they can also serve as reminders and triggers of the loss and trauma that you just experienced.

ACQUAINTANCES. Someone who has not experienced a reproductive loss might not understand why sharing the news with acquaintances is so daunting. After all, if they are just acquaintances, why does it matter what they think?

Time and again, women who have experienced a reproductive loss have expressed grave concern about encountering acquaintances who knew they were pregnant and who they only see from time to time. They imagine that the scenario will go like this: They will encounter the acquaintance at random; the acquaintance will ask about their pregnancy (or express confusion if it appears as if they are no longer pregnant, but the timing is not right for that to be the case); there will be an awkward moment when they have to share the news with the acquaintance; they fall apart, either right there in front of the acquaintance or immediately thereafter; and they experience the awful aftereffects of falling apart for the next several hours.

Some readers may find it helpful to have a general response prepared in advance to rely on in these sorts of instances. Only you can know what is right for you to communicate, specifically. Some people just say straightforwardly that the pregnancy didn't work out. Others say that the pregnancy didn't work out and then indicate how they are doing, for example, "It's a tough time, but we're surviving." Still others say that the pregnancy didn't work out and then attempt to redirect the conversation, such as, "Tell me how you are doing." Remember that you are under no obligation to provide additional detail or disclose your reproductive plans for the future unless you'd like to do so. In my experience, most acquaintances are thoughtful and supportive in their responses. A few might say things that are meant to be helpful but that can nonetheless sting (e.g., "Boy, it's always the ones who want children the most who can't have them"). Just remember that the acquaintances are trying, in their own way, to be supportive, and that you can exit the conversation at the first opportunity. In the rare instance in which an acquaintance inappropriately asks questions that you are not ready to answer, you have every right to respond assertively with a statement such as, "I truly appreciate your concern. Right now, I'm just not comfortable talking about it in more detail. I hope you understand that I'm still trying to figure all of this out."

Men's Perspective on Sharing the News. Men also encounter the same sorts of challenges as women do in telling family, friends, colleagues, clients, and acquaintances who knew about the pregnancy. It is true that it will not be obvious from their bodies that a loss occurred. However, people who knew about the pregnancy may well ask about it.

On the other hand, men face some unique issues regarding the sharing of news of the loss with others. As one male client stated to me, "Unless there is a specific reason to do so, men don't go around announcing the pregnancy to their buddies." Thus, when a loss occurs, they are clearly affected by it, but the source of the upset will not be obvious to others. As my client stated, "I'm just walking around being quiet and mopey, and people are wondering, 'Hey, what's wrong with him?'" This kind of scenario contributes to perception sometimes reported by men whose female partners have experienced a reproductive loss—that their own suffering is invisible.

Men sometimes find that the simplest question—"How are you?"—takes on profound meaning in the time following a reproductive loss. Does one respond with the traditional "fine" so as not to get into the details? Or does one truly share how he is doing? As I stated in the previous sections of this chapter, men can choose any way to respond to this question they see fit—there is no right or wrong way to approach this seemingly innocuous question. The male client described in the previous paragraph had a prepared way of handling this question. Rather than responding with "I'm fine," he responded with, "I'm hanging in there." If the recipient of this response did not probe further, my client left it at that. However, if the recipient of this response asked further questions (e.g., "Hey, is everything alright?"), my client answered with a response like, "We recently experienced a family tragedy, so we're just trying to take care of ourselves right now and get back on our feet." With such a response, this client believed that he was honoring his grief without going into excessive detail with an acquaintance or old friend.

Addressing Others Who "Say the Wrong Thing"

There will be times when well-meaning people will say something about the reproductive loss that will seem inaccurate, insensitive, or dismissive. I have never encountered an instance in which the person making such a remark was intentionally trying to say something hurtful. Rather, it was more the case that the person blurted something out without truly considering the impact it would have on the person who experienced the loss. Here is a sampling of some reactions to the loss that have the potential to rub you the wrong way:

- "Everything happens for a reason."
- "It's God's will."
- "You just need to move on and try again."
- "Think of how much worse this would be if you lost a child when he or she was older."
- "I experienced a loss before—I know exactly how you're feeling" (when, in truth, the nature of the person's loss was very different than your loss).
- "You can just adopt."
- "Some people aren't meant to be parents."
- [if relevant] "You're young; you'll get pregnant again."
- [if relevant] "At least you have a child."

The fundamental issues with many of these and other responses to the loss are that such responses suggest that the other (a) knows exactly what you're feeling, (b) knows what is best in this situation, and (c) believes that he or she is pointing out something that "should" make you feel better and put things in perspective. There is no question that these types of comments can feel inappropriate, irritating, and hurtful. Remember that you can apply the thought modification strategies described in Chapters 4 and 5 of this book to evaluate the larger picture associated with these statements. If you conclude that the person making these statements is insensitive and unhelpful, it is likely that you will close that person off from your support network at a time when you need your support network the most. If you conclude that the person made an untimely remark, but that he or she was meaning to help, it is likely that you will continue to include that person in your support network. Asking yourself the question "What explanations might account for the reason why this person made this statement?" might help you to keep the comment in perspective.

It's up to you whether you want to take issue with one of these types of statements. You certainly have the right to respond accordingly if somebody says something offensive to you. However, you also might want to ensure that you are thinking clearly about doing what is "right" versus what is "effective." In other words, are there any costs to you if you do take issue with the person's comment? One result might be that you close that person off from your social support network. It might well be that the person is not contributing helpful support and would be better off being outside of your support network, but I encourage you to make that decision in a thoughtful manner. Another result might be that it exacerbates your emotional pain at a difficult time. Thus, even if you are upset by a comment, it might be in your best interest to let it go for your own emotional well-being after the reproductive loss.

On the other hand, you might choose to respond to people who make insensitive comments about the reproductive loss. I've heard many reasons why people who have experienced reproductive loss choose to respond, including (a) it honors the grief that they are experiencing and their unborn child; (b) it educates the other about reproductive loss; and (c) it is a way to take care of themselves because they anticipate that, otherwise, they would stew and ruminate over the comment. If you do choose to respond to a comment that you perceive as insensitive, I would encourage you to be mindful of two principles. The first principle is *Choose your battles wisely*—you want to ensure that you are not taking on so many "battles" that it is taking valuable energy away from your capacity to achieve healing and growth from this experience. The second principle encompasses the components of assertiveness described earlier in this chapter.

Think about what is common among the assertive responses that I have described in the chapter to this point. First, they usually begin with a statement that either acknowledges the other's point of view or gives the person the benefit of the doubt that their comments are made out of care and concern. Second, they clearly describe a request. And third, they often provide a statement that either provides positive reinforcement or that provides further rationale for the request without being overly apologetic, on the one hand, or aggressive, on the other hand. All the while, these assertive statements are made with a calm, even tone of voice and appropriate nonverbal behavior that is commensurate with the message that is being communicated. An example, then, of a response that could be made to an insensitive remark is, "I appreciate that you're expressing care and concern by trying to help me move past this. One thing I've learned, though, is that there is no right or wrong way to view a reproductive loss. I think I'm experiencing this in a different way than you might experience it, and that I need to make sense of this at my own pace."

Fielding Questions About Childbearing

As time goes on, you may find that others ask you about trying again. These questions can trigger all sorts of worries and anxieties—many of which were captured in the "what-if" questions described in Chapter 5. Moreover, these questions can reopen old wounds if you are having trouble getting pregnant, are going through time-consuming fertility treatments, or have decided that it is in your best interest to stop trying.

There are many ways to field questions about having children in the future. Some people choose to share a vague response, such as, "We'll just have to see what happens." Other people will share a direct statement, such as, "We've decided to keep our family the size that it is." Still other people decide that drawing boundaries about topics that are and are not OK to talk about are in order, particularly if the person asking the question is not a family member or close friend. In these instances, an assertive response could be something like, "I appreciate your interest in my well-being. However, there are a lot of pieces to this issue that make it complicated."

In my experience, parents who have one child seem to get bombarded with even more questions about future childbearing than adults who do not have children. I suspect that these questions arise from people's observations that many couples try to have children that are 2 or 3 years apart in age, as well as from the stereotype that single children (a term I prefer over "only children") are somehow at a social and emotional disadvantage relative to children with siblings. It can be painful to hear over and over again, "When are you going to give your child a little sister or brother?" for a number of reasons: (a) It was so difficult for you to conceive or carry a single child or (b) you have been investing a great deal of time, energy, and resources into having another child, and it does not seem to be happening. Responses that you can consider in these circumstances include the following:

- "Thanks for asking, but we're just fine as we are."
- "Thanks for asking, but we consider ourselves a terrific and fortunate family with one child."
- "Thanks for asking, but we find that families come in all shapes and sizes, and there is no one size fits all."
- "Whatever happens, happens, but in the meantime we're thoroughly enjoying the child we do have."

Although it is unfortunate, at times a person may express a definite negative opinion about having a single child. Often, people who express these opinions are the same ones who have opinions about many aspects of childbearing—the acceptability of fertility treatments, how best to take care of oneself during pregnancy, how best to sleep-train or potty-train a child, and so on. These people may give you the message that by having a single child, you are setting up that child to be spoiled, socially unskilled, lonely, and moody. Fortunately, research summarized by psychologist Susan Newman has shown that none of these concerns are valid—that single children are similar to children with siblings in a host of personality traits and life outcomes. In fact, some research even suggests that single children are closer to their parents (in a healthy manner) than children who have siblings, which is a finding that has the potential to be heartening for parents who are able to have only one child. Responses to people who express negative opinions about having one child can include the following:

- "Thanks for your concern, but there are a number of factors that have gone into our decision, and we're quite comfortable with it."
- "Thanks for your concern, but we've done our research on this topic, and research shows that single children will be just fine."
- "Thanks for your concern, but we feel blessed to have a child and are committed to being the best parents we can be."
- "Thanks for your concern, but we find that families come in all shapes and sizes, and there is no one size fits all."

Interacting With Expectant Parents

We have already discussed interactions with expectant parents with whom you are friends at the time of a reproductive loss. However, it is an unfortunate reality that you will continue to be exposed to expectant parents—friends, colleagues, clients, acquaintances, and strangers that you meet randomly—throughout your life, and especially when you are of childbearing age. You might feel some "sting" in these interactions for months and even years to come. I say more in Chapter 7 about gradually resuming contact with expectant parents at a pace that you can handle. Here, I consider ways of handling interactions with expectant parents.

One rule of thumb to keep in mind is that short, simple statements of congratulations or that express some other type of support usually suffice. If someone tells you that she is expecting, you can say something like, "Congratulations, that is terrific news" without asking for excessive detail. If someone tells you a funny story about his son, you can say something like, "Your son sounds precious, enjoy these moments with him" without asking for additional pieces of the story. If someone is complaining about her child, you can something like, "It sounds like your daughter has been frustrating you lately" without asking for more detail or reminding her that she is fortunate to have a child. The philosophy underlying the rule of thumb of staying simple is that you are doing what is effective in simultaneously maintaining relationships and taking care of yourself as you continue to process your grief.

However, if you would like to ask about details and engage in more conversation about others' pregnancies or children, by all means do so. Being involved in the lives of friends and their children can certainly bring a sense of happiness and belonging.

Interacting With People From the Past

Encounters with people from your past can be difficult because one of the questions that invariably arises as you are catching up with one another is, "Do you have children?" If you're struggling with infertility, then it is excruciating to respond "no" to this question.

If you have experienced a miscarriage, neonatal loss, stillbirth, or death of a very young child, do you acknowledge this? In the latter scenario, some people find that it is most effective simply not to acknowledge the child that had been lost so as not to prompt additional questions (or so that your loss does not become public knowledge to others from your past if you do not want it to be public). However, others feel strongly that acknowledging the loss is a way to honor the child. You have every right to choose whatever route is best for you. Whatever you decide, I recommend that you think ahead of time about the type of assertive response you'd like to give so that you are prepared.

Requesting Special Accommodations

Anyone who has undergone fertility treatments knows that they are extremely time-consuming and sometimes require you to drop everything and attend an appointment with your fertility doctor at key times in your cycle. This would be stressful for almost anyone, and if you are expected to be at work at a prescribed time each day, it can seem impossible to negotiate. If you are not in control of your own schedule, you might find yourself in a situation in which you will need to let someone at work (e.g., supervisor, business administrator) know what is happening to request time off. It can feel awkward to be sharing intimate details about your reproductive health with a colleague or coworker with whom you otherwise would not have a relationship.

Only you can decide how much background information is appropriate to share with a supervisor or business administrator who will grant you flexibility and time off for fertility appointments. Many women find that sharing at least a small bit of information is helpful in order to provide a context for their colleague to grant the request. You might reference, specifically, that you are undergoing fertility treatment, or you might indicate, more generally, that you are underling ongoing medical tests or procedures. In addition to requesting time off for these appointments, you might also be faced with arranging for a coworker to cover your shift or some of your duties, and the same question concerning the amount of information to communicate will likely arise. In all of these instances, the principles of assertive communication are relevant—provide a bit of context, make the request, and follow with positive reinforcement.

You might consider preparing for some questions posed by others that you experience as intrusive. Perhaps your colleagues ask for more detail. Perhaps they check in and ask how your appointments went. By thinking in advance how to field these questions, the likelihood that you will be caught off guard is minimized. In addition, depending on the culture of your work setting, you may want to think about how public you want your situation to be. If your work environment is one that falls prey to gossip, it might behoove you to ask your colleagues who know about your situation to keep any of your discussions confidential.

CONNECTING WITH YOUR SPOUSE OR PARTNER

It is logical to expect your spouse or partner to have the most intricate understanding of your state following a reproductive loss because, after all, he or she experienced the loss, too. Some couples find great comfort in one another following a loss. However, other couples find that they feel disconnected from one another. In this section, I consider different reasons why you may feel disconnected from your spouse or partner, as well as ways to maintain and enhance the relationship during this difficult time.

Your Spouse or Partner Has a Different Style of Grieving

Incongruous grief is one of the most common concerns expressed by people who have experienced reproductive loss. In heterosexual couples, it often is the case (but certainly not always) that the male partner addresses the loss by problem solving ways to overcome fertility problems, by externalizing his emotions and delving into other activities (e.g., work, sports), or by simply willing himself to "move on." In contrast, it is often (but certainly not always) the case that the female partner addresses the loss by emotional experiencing, creating memoirs of the lost child and talking about the loss with others. Interestingly, female partners may engage in just as much, if not more, problem solving to overcome fertility problems as male partners do, although sometimes it "feels" different because having child is often more intricately related to a woman's self-esteem than it is to a man's self-esteem. Indeed, sociologist Arthur Greil's work suggests that it might seem that male partners approach the problem in a manner in which they would solve any problems that they encounter, whereas women approach the problem as a threat to their identities.

Of course, these are generalizations, and I don't want to emphasize gender stereotypes. There are plenty of heterosexual couples in whom the nature of the grieving process is reversed, and there are plenty of homosexual couples in whom each member may or may not process grief according to traditional gender roles. Nevertheless, the fact remains that many couples find that each individual grieves in a different manner—something they would not have expected or realized when they first entered into their committed relationship—and that these different styles leave one another feeling baffled, and perhaps even unsupported and disconnected. Such differences don't have to cause a rift in the marriage or relationship, but it's important to recognize and respect these differences to minimize violated expectations and miscommunication and to find a middle ground in which both partners' needs are being met.

One Spouse or Partner Feels a Need to Take Care of the Other Spouse or Partner

In many (but not all) cases, the spouse or partner who was not carrying the child believes that he or she needs to be strong for the person who was carrying the child. The male client whom I mentioned earlier in this chapter believed that he needed to do everything he could to take care of his wife who delivered a stillborn child near full term, including fully caring for their older daughter (i.e., getting her ready for school, feeding her, preparing her lunch, playing with her on evenings and weekends, bathing her, putting her to bed), doing all of the household errands and chores, and "being there" to soothe his wife. In doing so, others observed that he was not taking time to address his own grief. Although this man did not feel disconnected from his wife (and was determined not to let the loss tear them apart), he recognized that he might not be able to go on like this forever. It was at that point that he entered into individual therapy to manage his own grief so that he could maintain fulfilling relationships with his wife and daughter.

Your Spouse or Partner Has Different Childbearing Goals

A reproductive loss can spur different types of action in each spouse or partner. One spouse or partner may decide to do everything possible to have a child, and the other spouse or partner may decide that he or she has had enough. Spouses and partners can disagree on a host of different fertility-related issues, such as (a) whether to proceed with infertility treatments, (b) whether to use a donor egg or donor sperm, (c) the amount of money to spend on fertility treatments, and (d) whether to proceed with adoption. If they become pregnant again, they might disagree on aspects of prenatal care, such as whether to have an amniocentesis.

What's difficult about these issues is that most couples do not anticipate that they will be in a position in which they are faced with these decisions, so they have not discussed in advance where they stand on these issues. Even if they have discussed these issues in advance, in the aftermath of a reproductive loss, one or both spouses or partners might change their stances. The couple finds themselves, then, in a position in which the person who does not "get his or her way" might view the other person as being the gatekeeper to having a child and become resentful. This resentment could spread into other areas of the relationship that were once strong and fulfilling.

What to Do About a Disconnect With Your Partner

There is no magic pill that will make a relationship feel more connected after a reproductive loss, and there is no question that rebuilding a close, connected, relationship takes time and devotion. However, communication is key. Giving one another the cold shoulder, avoiding one another, or throwing yourself into other activities without your partner will only serve to widen the chasm. You may not always like what your partner has to say, and your partner may not always like what you have to say. However, if you communicate openly, honestly, and respectfully, remembering the love that brought you together in the first place, you will begin to repair that disconnect so that you can provide one another the support that you need as you cope with the reproductive loss. The following are some specific suggestions for repairing the disconnect:

- *Be explicit about your style of grieving.* It is easy for your spouse or partner to misinterpret your grieving behavior as being something other than what it is. For example, if you tend to avoid reminders of the loss, your spouse or partner might misinterpret that as not caring as much as he or she does. Clarifying the manner in which you grieve is a way to promote understanding in your spouse or partner.

- *Understand that there is no one way to grieve a reproductive loss.* It is OK for your spouse or partner to be grieving in a different manner than you are, and it is important to be respectful of that. At times, you may even feel uncomfortable with your spouse or partner's style of grieving. In this instance, it will be important to strike a balance between making requests to get your own needs met while respecting and even tolerating your spouse or partner's way of grieving.

- *Clarify your assumptions about your spouse or partner's behavior.* I find that much of couples' miscommunication stems from one spouse's or partner's making an (incorrect) assumption about the reasons that underlie the other spouse or partner's behavior. One approach would be to say something like, "When you say _____, I take it as _____. Is this what you are intending? Or am I misreading something?" Such communication helps to get assumptions on the table and ensure that both parties are crystal clear on the motivations and expectations that underlie their behavior.

- *Adopt a relationship-focused problem orientation.* A *problem orientation* refers to the cognitive set that people bring to a problem, disagreement, or conflict. Differences of opinion between spouses or partners about their reproductive futures can become highly charged, often resulting in each party adopting a self-focused problem orientation, such that each party wants to solve the problem his or her way at all costs. By joining together and reorienting yourselves so that you can address the problem in light of what's good for the relationship, you can move toward reclaiming the teamwork relationship that you once had and work with, rather than against, each other. Of course, this is easier said than done when each party is tied closely to the solution that he or she so desperately wants. It will be important to be mindful that the ultimate solution will likely be a compromise. Moreover, it will also be important for each party to fully commit to and implement his or her part of the solution that is decided on.

- *Use a calm, even voice.* I mentioned the calm, even voice earlier in the chapter, and nowhere is it more important to use a calm, even voice than in addressing disconnect in one's partner relationship. From a practical standpoint, use of a calm, even voice prevents disagreements from escalating, which so easily happens in partner relational disagreements. However, the calm, even voice also communicates a tone of respect for the other person's viewpoint and a willingness to listen. All of these factors increase the likelihood that the relationship disconnect will begin to be repaired and that any problems that need to be addressed be solved.

- *Remember the key points of assertive communication.* All of the points of assertive communication that have been reinforced throughout this chapter apply to repair of partner relationship disconnect. Specifically, first acknowledging the other person's point of view when making a request can make a world of difference in promoting a context of respect and collaboration. Moreover, providing a rationale for specific requests you are making will help your partner to understand where you are coming from and has the potential to provide important information that he or she otherwise would not have had. Conversely, watch out so that you do not fall into an aggressive, passive, or passive–aggressive communication style that might thwart your efforts to achieve connection in your relationship. You and your spouse or partner are already feeling vulnerable following the reproductive loss, and it is important to behave in a caring manner in light of that vulnerability, rather than in a way that entrenches it further.

- *Refrain from fighting unfairly.* Many experts on relationships and couples therapy define "fighting fairly" differently, but here I focus on two main sets of behaviors that can quickly thwart communication. One set involves bringing in "baggage" from the past. Remember that the issue at hand is the disconnect in the relationship that has arisen from the tremendous loss that you and your spouse or partner experienced. The two of you obviously have a history together, and it is easy in times of hurt and vulnerability to remember old wounds that you inflicted on one another. The two of you have a formidable task ahead in supporting one another as you grieve the reproductive loss, and now is not the time to complicate the issue. The second set of behaviors involves what has been termed by renowned relationships scholar Dr. John Gottman as character assassination. *Character assassination* refers to the tendency to speak negatively about the character of the other. Examples include "You are selfish and always think of yourself" and "You're so weak that you break down when the slightest thing happens." When you find yourself using language that includes the words "you always" or "you never," or when you find yourself pinning negative personality traits on your spouse or partner, then you are engaging in character assassination. Extreme examples of character assassination are name-calling and hurling below-the-belt insults. Character assassination clearly is not productive because it puts the other on the defensive, which moves you further away from solving your problem. Moreover, it creates an unsafe environment for your spouse or partner to share his or her vulnerability.

- *Engage in behaviors that facilitate a sense of connection.* Although open and effective communication is vitally important for improving connection with your spouse or partner, it is also important to engage in other behaviors consistent with connection and closeness. Recall Karen from Chapter 5, who was feeling disconnected from her partner and identified a number of things she could do to repair the connection, such as a weekly date night. Implementation of effective communication skills will help you "talk the talk" of relationship repair; implementation of shared activities (especially those that are pleasurable or meaningful in your relationship) will help you "walk the walk." Ways to walk the walk include physical closeness (not necessarily sex), engaging in a shared activity that both of you used to enjoy, and going away for a long weekend.

UTILIZING YOUR SUPPORT NETWORK

I include a section on utilizing your social support network in this chapter because doing so requires that you interact with others in that network. The reason I view this as so important is that positive social support from others is known to be a buffer against depression, anxiety, and other emotional upset. Positive social support can mean a lot of things, such as the provision of a nonjudgmental, listening ear or the provision of information and resources. When a person perceives that she is receiving positive social support from others in her support network, it means that she views that support as helpful.

Recall that, in Chapter 2, I suggested that you reach out to at least one person even if it is just for a brief cup of coffee or to spend a couple of hours in one of your homes. The rationale behind this suggestion was for you to obtain some social support, which would in turn help you begin the process of grieving and making sense of your reproductive loss. Over time, and when you are ready, you can widen your circle and increase the degree to which you utilize your social support network. It will seem like a lot of effort, and you might not be sure if it is worth it. You might have to pick and choose whom you will include in your expanded circle, depending on whether some of these other are pregnant, have small children, or were less helpful than you had anticipated in the immediate aftermath of the reproductive loss. However, in the long run, doing so will help you to feel connected to others, and perhaps more generally to your life itself. It will help to direct your attention to something other than the loss. And it will remind you that people love you and care for your well-being, which will foster a sense of community at a time when it feels like you are so alone.

Although to this point in this section, I have been focusing on positive social support, I should also acknowledge that there are times when you will experience negative social support from others. *Negative social support* is an attempt by another person to give you some sort of support that you experience as unhelpful or aversive and that can exacerbate your experience of depression, anxiety, or emotional upset. Thus, if you are experiencing expressions of support as unhelpful, you have every right to exercise the limits and draw the boundaries that I described earlier in this chapter. Down the line, you might see that the person's efforts were well intended and perhaps even right on target. But if you're not ready to accept them, you're not ready.

THE ULTIMATE GOAL: TAKING CARE OF YOURSELF

Assertive communication works because it maximizes the likelihood that you will achieve your desired aims—you make a request of others, you say no to others, you define limits and boundaries, and so on. You are clearly stating what you desire. At the same time, you are respecting that others might have a different viewpoint, and you acknowledge that outright. Using this communication style with others shows that you understand that they have a viewpoint and invites them into a dialogue, as opposed to backing them into a corner, such that the likelihood of a defensive response increases.

Using assertive communication specifically after a reproductive loss works because you are taking care of yourself first, rather than accommodating others or behaving according to what others think you "should" be doing. I firmly believe that it also has the potential to preserve relationships, especially relationships with family members, friends, and coworkers who are pregnant or who have small children. You simply might not be able to be in their presence for a while, and although they almost assuredly will understand, over time it can affect the relationship. Letting these people in on exactly where you are in the grieving process, as well as expressing to them that you care about them, can go a long way in getting the space you need and allowing you to resume the relationship when you are ready.

Many of the examples in this chapter describe ways to let others know you need space. In my experience, this is the most common need stated by people who have experienced a reproductive loss. However, you might find yourself with a different set of needs—to share your experience and to show your emotion. It can be therapeutic to talk about your loss with someone who shows genuine concern. There may be tears. But this sharing has the potential to help you to process your grief while enhancing a relationship with someone who cares about you.

CHAPTER 7

GRADUAL EXPOSURE TO AVOIDED SITUATIONS

I have stated multiple times throughout this book that it is difficult for people who have experienced reproductive loss and trauma to be in the presence of pregnant women, infants, and young children. Countless people have described the great lengths to which they have gone to avoid social gatherings, parks, stores, and especially events such as children's birthday parties, baby showers, and baptisms. If this describes you, know that you are not alone. If your loss is recent, it's understandable that you are doing what you need to do to get by and that being in the presence of a reminder of the loss is just too triggering. Over time, however, avoidance can backfire and actually increase the intensity of your emotional distress. In this chapter, I describe exactly why this can happen and how you can overcome it.

THE VICIOUS CYCLE

When you are upset, it is natural that you would want to take measures to feel better. And when something reminds you of a painful time in your life, it is natural to do what you can to get rid of that reminder. When you get rid of a reminder of a painful time in your life, it gives you a temporary sense of relief, or at least a decrease in

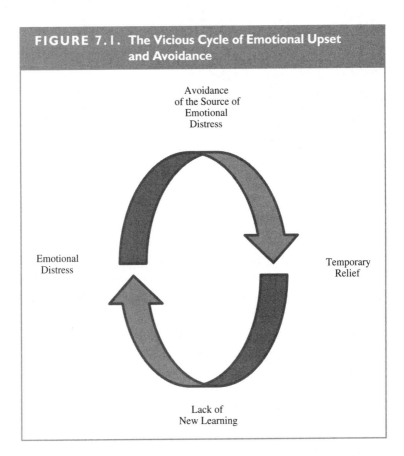

FIGURE 7.1. The Vicious Cycle of Emotional Upset and Avoidance

the intensity of your emotional upset. However, this reinforces the avoidance behavior by the removing an aversive emotional state. Figure 7.1 depicts this vicious cycle. The more you avoid, the more avoidance is reinforced by the decrease in the intensity of emotional upset, which in turn increases the likelihood of avoidance in the future. In addition, the dread of and aversion to future encounters with reminders of painful times in your life increase exponentially because you have not learned that you can handle them. In other words, when you avoid reminders of the loss, you get a temporary decrease in emotional distress, but dread and aversion boomerang back at you.

The way to break out of this vicious cycle is to begin to have contact with the very reminders and triggers that you are avoiding. The technical term for this process is *exposure*. I realize this sounds awful and like the last thing you want to do. However, if you find that avoidance behavior, dread, and aversion toward encounters with reminders of the loss are taking over more and more facets of your life, you might consider gradually reengaging with the world, such that you come in contact with these reminders and show yourself that you can, indeed, tolerate them and cope with them. I mentioned exposure briefly in Chapter 4 as it related to overcoming avoidance of intrusive thoughts that are incompletely processed. Here I focus on exposure to contact with external stimuli (e.g., places, people, and other reminders of the loss or trauma). The principles underlying both types of exposure are the same, however.

Many people who have experienced a reproductive loss believe that having contact with a reminder of young children will be intolerable, and they worry about breaking down, going into a terrible funk, or going crazy. Exposure gives you the opportunity to learn something different. You learn that you *can* cope. You learn that you *can* tolerate the intense emotion. You learn that the awful outcome you had expected did not occur. You learn that you might even have some emotional experiences that are mildly pleasant. Think back to the thinking traps that were presented in Chapters 4 and 5. You might have some predictions of what you think will occur when you have contact with a trigger or a reminder of the loss that is consistent with some of those thinking traps (e.g., fortune-telling, catastrophizing, all-or-nothing thinking). Engaging in exposure is a way of testing those out, and if the worst-case outcome does not occur, then you have gained important information that can guide your behavior in future encounters with reminders of your loss. If you avoid, then you are not able to capitalize on this new learning.

Exposure is not an easy process. It takes a consistent effort, and most people experience a temporary increase in emotional distress when they have contact with the triggers and reminders they have been avoiding. It is important, then, to think about the benefits that exposure can bring you because focusing on these benefits will provide much-needed motivation when the avoidance pattern seems too great to overcome. Are you avoiding certain friends and family members who are an important part of your social support network? Are you isolating yourself at home, getting out much less than you used to? Are you spending a lot of time planning errands and other outings for times you would be unlikely to run into a reminder of your loss? Or are you simply filled with dread, just awaiting the next reminder? Most important, is it in your best interest to live this way?

The bottom line is that living a life motivated primarily by avoidance will likely deprive you of the opportunities you need to actively engage in life and obtain the benefits described in Chapters 2 and 3. Practicing exposure to the triggers and reminders that you encounter in everyday life will help you shift away from an avoidance orientation and toward an approach orientation, or an orientation in which you live a life that is consistent with your values.

WHERE DO I START?

I can appreciate that this process seems daunting and that it's easier said than done. Please know that you can go at your own pace. If you feel forced to go through this process, it will be less effective than if you commit to it because it's important to you.

The basic idea that underlies exposure is that you start small and work your way up to contact with increasingly difficult triggers and reminders of the loss. Once you have developed mastery over a small trigger or reminder, you then turn your attention to a more difficult trigger or reminder. You can arrange the triggers and reminders from least to most difficult using a tool called a *hierarchy*. The following steps can guide you in developing your own personalized hierarchy.

1. Brainstorm the full pool of situations, events, and places that you are avoiding because you might encounter a trigger or a reminder of the loss.
2. Rate the level of emotional upset or dread associated with each situation, event, or place on a 10-point scale (0 = *the absence of emotional upset or dread*; 10 = *the most emotional upset or dread that you can imagine*).
3. Order the situations, events, and places, starting with the item associated with the lowest level of emotional upset or dread and ending with the item associated with the highest level of emotional upset or dread.

Remember Kristin from Chapter 2, who was depressed in the period after her reproductive loss and was focused on what she could do to get out of bed. Over time, she reengaged in many of her usual activities, but she found that she was taking great pains to avoid encounters with pregnant women and infants. She decided to pursue gradual exposure when she was invited to her cousin's baby shower. She believed that she would greatly disappoint her close-knit family if she chose not to attend the shower, but at the same time, she was already consumed by dread, and it was still many weeks away. She resolved to devote the weeks preceding the shower to practice being in the presence of pregnant women and young children. The first thing she did was develop a hierarchy to guide her (see Figure 7.2).

One notable feature of Kristin's hierarchy is that it is creative: It incorporates places to go (e.g., grocery store, children's clothing

FIGURE 7.2. Kristin's Hierarchy

1. Shop at grocery store. (2)
2. Have lunch with friend who has a 6-year-old child. (3)
3. Go to a party where there will be a few children in attendance. (4)
4. Drive by elementary school on a weekend. (5)
5. Watch a movie about a family with children. (6)
6. Have lunch with friend who has a 2-year-old child. (7.5)
7. Go into a children's clothing store. (9)
8. Drive by an elementary school when the kids are arriving. (9)
9. Sit on a bench and watch the kids at the neighborhood park. (9.5)
10. Attend baby shower. (10)

store), places to observe children (e.g., school, neighborhood park), interactions with others who have children of different ages, and movies to watch. Notice that some of the items are similar and represent different manifestations of the same theme. For example, when she was developing her hierarchy, Kristin recognized that driving by a school would be difficult for her, and she could not imagine how she could bring herself to do such a thing. However, she realized that driving by the school would trigger different amounts of dread depending on when she drove by. She expected that she would not see any children at the school if she were to drive by during a weekend, whereas she would see many children if she drove by in the morning at a time when they would be dropped off for school. Not surprisingly, Kristin estimated that she would experience less dread and emotional upset if she drove past the school on the weekend, relative to a weekday morning. She viewed driving past the school on the weekend as a stepping-stone to driving past the school during the week when children were arriving. The timing of driving by the school was only one dimension that Kristin varied; she could have added other variations to her hierarchy as well. For example, she could have included driving by a variety of types of schools, such as a high school, a middle school, an elementary school, and a preschool, with the idea that the high school and middle school would be associated with less dread and emotional upset than the elementary school and preschool.

I have several tips that can make your hierarchy as effective and comprehensive as possible. First, typing your hierarchy into a computer document (e.g., a Microsoft Word or Excel table) often allows for the greatest amount of flexibility. Despite your best efforts, when you sit down to develop your hierarchy, you probably won't be able to think of every single trigger or reminder that you have been avoiding. You'll likely identify other situations, events, and places that you have been avoiding when you encounter them in your daily life. By having the items in an electronic file, you can easily add additional items at a later time in their proper place, on the basis of the intensity of dread that you rate. Second, try to include as many items as you can that you can replicate at any time. Notice the third item on Kristin's hierarchy: Go to a party where there will be a few children in attendance. Kristin included this item because she was anticipating a party to which she was invited that was taking place in approximately 2 weeks. However, it was something she could only practice when such an event was scheduled. Inclusion of some of these occasional events is OK because that's the way that life works, but make sure you include other items that you can accomplish at any time.

Keep in mind that the hierarchy does not have to include only situations, events, and places where you might run into pregnant women and young children. It can also include other reminders of the loss or trauma that you might be avoiding, such as the hospital, a place of worship, or your child's gravesite. If you believe that avoidance of these other reminders is interfering with your functioning or otherwise exacerbating your emotional distress, then by all means include them on your hierarchy. This is the approach Angela took; on her hierarchy, she included items such as speaking to her obstetrician, going into the main lobby of the hospital, and reading through the cards and e-mail messages sent from others when they learned of the loss. The rules of thumb that you can use when deciding what to include and what not to include on your hierarchy are as follows: (a) Is avoidance of this situation, event, or place causing interference in my life or exacerbating my emotional distress? (b) Will this be a situation, event, or place that I will encounter over and over, such that it would be in my best interest to learn to approach it rather than avoid it? and (c) Is avoiding this situation, event, or place inconsistent with my core values?

You might sit down to develop your hierarchy and realize that you don't exactly know what to include. That's OK; avoidance behavior is sometimes subtle, and sometimes we don't even recognize that we are setting up our lives in a way that perpetuates avoidance. If this is the case, it might help to engage in an activity called *self-monitoring*, which is a way for you to prospectively track situations in which you experience emotional upset or dread, associated features such as physiological reactions and negative thoughts, the behaviors in which you engage to reduce emotional upset or dread (especially avoidance), and the degree to which these coping skills are or are not effective. Figure 7.3 is an example of a self-monitoring form. The goal of self-monitoring is for you to notice, as you live your life, instances that trigger emotional distress, your internal reactions to them, and the degree to which your behavioral responses are actually helpful. Self-monitoring not only allows you to identify situations in which you exhibit either avoidance or escape behavior, it also gives you a sense of the thoughts that run through your mind in these situations. Those thoughts can be managed using the thought modification skills described in Chapters 4 and 5. This is an example of the fact that the strategies and tools described in this book are not

FIGURE 7.3. Self-Monitoring Form

Situation or Trigger	Emotion and Intensity	Physiological Reaction	Thought	Coping Behavior (Avoidance?)	Result of Coping Behavior

generally used in isolation; their combined application covers multiple angles of recovery and grieving after a reproductive loss.

IMPLEMENTING EXPOSURE

After you have developed your hierarchy, you will begin to implement the exposures in a systematic manner. Use your hierarchy as a guide to select the exposure you will do in any one instance. Although it is logical to start with the lowest rated item on the hierarchy and move up sequentially, research by psychologist Michelle Craske has shown that the most durable learning occurs when you attempt items on your hierarchy according to a random schedule.

Before beginning the exposure, rate your degree of confidence that you can tolerate the emotional distress associated with the exposure (0 = *no confidence*; 10 = *the highest level of confidence*). In addition, make a prediction as to the length of time you believe that you can tolerate the exposure, as well as any other predictions about bad things that you expect will happen during the exposure. Check in with yourself and make similar ratings periodically as you go through the exposure to see if your confidence level increases and to monitor whether any of your other negative predictions have been realized. Even if you are still experiencing a high level of emotional distress, you might see that your confidence levels increase throughout the exposure, and you might see that other negative outcomes you had anticipated have not occurred. You can exit the exposure when you remain in contact with the situation or stimulus for a longer period of time than you had originally predicted you would be able to do. Then make a final rating of your confidence that you can tolerate the emotional distress associated with the exposure. This procedure allows for new learning to occur because you will have shown yourself that you can tolerate being in the presence of dreaded stimuli and situations, and you will see that other aversive outcomes do not occur.

After you have completed the exposure, take time to reflect on your accomplishment. You have taken a big step to reengage with avoided situations and stimuli. If it did not go as planned or if you did not achieve the outcomes described in the previous paragraph, don't beat yourself up. Remember that this is a process; simply attempting this exercise means you are taking your recovery seriously. There will be other opportunities to practice.

It is important to engage in each exposure on more than one occasion. What you will likely see is that, with each subsequent practice, your ratings of confidence that you can tolerate emotional distress increase. In addition, you will have consolidated new learning, so that with each subsequent time you face the dreaded situation or stimulus, the likelihood increases that the new learning (e.g., "I can get through this") will be activated instead of the old fears (e.g., "I will break down and be in a funk for months"). Figure 7.4 is an example of an Exposure Recording Form on which you can track your progress, and Figure 7.5 displays an excerpt from Kristin's Exposure Rating Form. It is hoped that these "data" will give you some hope because you'll have a record of your hard work, and you'll see some changes in the cognitive orientation to which you bring to the exposure because of the new learning you have acquired. As a result, you will start to feel a bit more freedom in the kinds of activities in which you engage in your daily life.

Strive to include as much variability in your exposures as possible; recent research shows that practicing exposures in a number of environments and circumstances increases the generalization of its effects. For example, you will see on Kristin's Exposure Rating Form (Figure 7.5) that she practiced going to the grocery store on a number of occasions. Rather than shopping at the same store at the same time each week, she shopped at different stores at different times to maximize the likelihood that she would remember her new learning, wherever she might be. Moreover, Michelle Craske's research suggests

FIGURE 7.4. Exposure Recording Form

Date	Exposure	Confidence in Ability to Tolerate Emotional Distress (Pre)	Confidence in Ability to Tolerate Emotional Distress (Post)	Other Observations

FIGURE 7.5. Kristin's Exposure Recording Form

Date	Exposure	Confidence in Ability to Tolerate Emotional Distress (Pre)	Confidence in Ability to Tolerate Emotional Distress (Post)	Other Observations
4/15	Shop at grocery store	2	8	Wasn't as bad as I thought.
4/17	Shop at grocery store	3	6	Saw a baby, it was hard.
4/20	Shop at grocery store	6	8	Getting easier.
4/21	Have lunch with friend who has a 6-year-old	2	6	I thought I would break down, but I didn't.
4/22	Shop at grocery store	7	9	
4/23	Drive by elementary school (weekend)	1	5	I thought I would really lose it, but I didn't.
4/24	Watch movie about a family with children	2	7	I cried, but it wasn't awful.
4/25	Shop at grocery store	8	10	I'm not worried about this one anymore.

(continued)

FIGURE 7.5. Kristin's Exposure Recording Form
(*Continued*)

Date	Exposure	Confidence in Ability to Tolerate Emotional Distress (Pre)	Confidence in Ability to Tolerate Emotional Distress (Post)	Other Observations
4/28	Have lunch with friend who has a 6-year-old	3	8	I felt a bit wistful, but not like I would break down.
4/29	Shop at grocery store	10	10	
4/30	Shop at the mall on weekend	4	9	Contrary to what I expected, I hardly saw any children.
4/30	Go to party with children in attendance	2	9	I did it. I'm glad I practiced the other exposures leading up to this one.

that the combination of exposure targets facilitates even more powerful learning than exposure to a single target. Thus, after several weeks of practicing her exposures, Kristin combined some of the items, such that she would have lunch with a friend who had children and then, with that friend, see a movie about a family with children.

There will undoubtedly be occasions when you are faced with an unexpected opportunity to approach (rather than avoid) a trigger or reminder of your reproductive loss that you otherwise would have avoidance. Such an instance is called a *lifestyle exposure*. Take another look at Kristin's Exposure Recording Form in Figure 7.5 and notice that one of the exposures she recorded was shopping at the mall on the weekend. Technically, this was not an item she had included on her hierarchy. However, she realized she had been avoiding shopping for a gift for the party she was attending the next day because she anticipated that she would encounter a plethora of babies and young children at the shopping mall. Rather than avoiding (e.g., ordering a gift online), she decided to seize the opportunity for an additional exposure and go to the mall. I encourage you to keep in mind the principles of exposure and take advantage of additional opportunities that arise in your daily life.

TROUBLESHOOTING: IT'S NOT WORKING

It's not uncommon for people to say they have tried exposure but continue to experience a great deal of emotional intensity that seems intolerable to them the next time they are faced with a trigger. When this occurs, the first thing for which you should be on the lookout is any safety behavior you might be using. A *safety behavior* is a subtle maneuver you might perform to reduce your level of emotional distress. For example, you might silently pray to yourself as you are doing the exposure; you might perform a mental ritual that is comforting, like counting by threes; or you might ask someone several times for reassurance that you can get through the exposure. You might even believe that you need to have another person accompany you when you are doing the exposure. There are two problems with safety behaviors. First, they prevent you from fully experiencing the emotional upset and dread, which does not allow you to learn that you can tolerate emotional distress on your own. Second, you create a situation in which it is easy to conclude that the only reason you got through the exposure was because you engaged in the behavior. Thus, although it might seem like these behaviors and maneuvers facilitate the exposure, they actually interfere with your ability to gain maximum benefit from it.

Safety behaviors are hard to give up. It could be that the only way you'd even consider doing an exposure is to engage in one of these behaviors. It is true that the goal of these exposures is to fully engage in the exercises without engaging in any competing safety behaviors. However, if using the safety behaviors will help you overcome the hurdle of simply engaging in the activity, use it the first time you engage in the exposure, and then work toward eliminating the safety behavior.

Another thing to remember is that you can use the other strategies and tools described in this book to cope effectively with the distress you experience in the exposure. Thought modification is a great example. If you have the idea "This is going to drive me insane. I'm going to be carted off to the hospital in a straitjacket," you can use your thought modification questions to get some distance and balance. You might construct a balanced response such as, "There is no doubt that this will be difficult. But I'll be able to handle it because I'm slowly working up to my most dreaded situations. I can take it at my own pace and practice my coping skills as I do the exposures."

Finally, I would encourage you to keep trying, perhaps even trying every day. Exposure is easy to put off because no one likes to be emotionally upset. However, putting it off is another form of avoidance, which only entrenches your anticipation of emotional upset and dread even further. I've had clients do one exposure a week and experience a significant amount of relief the other 6 days of the week—"Phew! That's over. I don't have to do that again for a while." To be effective, exposure needs to be done on a regular basis—every day if at all possible. Because exposure can use a great deal of your psychological coping resources, when you have completed the exercise, I would encourage you to do something to replenish those resources so that they are available the next day. Look forward to doing something pleasurable and enjoyable. Connect with a trusted member of your social support network. Take care of yourself. Once you have had success with sustained practice, you can begin to space out your attempts at exposure, which will help to solidify the long-term retention of your new learning.

HOPE FOR THE FUTURE

The research literature shows, without question, that exposure is highly effective in reducing emotional distress. However, as I have indicated throughout this chapter, it is also understandable that you will have some trepidation as you think about embarking on a schedule of exposure exercises. You *will* experience emotional upset. Keep in mind a phrase used by exposure expert Jonathan Abramowitz: "Invest in anxiety now for a calmer future." Translated to your situation, this means that if you invest the time and energy now to overcome avoidance of triggers and other reminders of the loss, you will be able to reclaim parts of your life to which you currently have little access. Many people who experience a reproductive loss find themselves feeling extraordinarily bitter and jealous when they are faced with a reminder of the reproductive loss, which is upsetting because it is wholly inconsistent with the manner in which they view themselves. Gradual exposure to these situations and triggers will help your body and mind adapt to those aversive emotional experiences, demonstrate that you can get through them with grace and dignity, and allow you to fully engage in many aspects of your life without investing mental energy into worrying about whether you will encounter a reminder of the reproductive loss. There is no question that it is hard work. But the outcome will allow you to fully grieve your loss and set yourself up to gain fulfillment and satisfaction from other things that life has to offer.

CHAPTER 8

PROBLEM SOLVING AND DECISION MAKING

People who have experienced reproductive loss face decisions at many junctures. Some decisions need to be made immediately after the loss, such as how to tell others of the loss and whether to have a funeral. Other decisions come later, such as whether to try to get pregnant again, whether to have children through different means (e.g., adoption), or whether to have medical procedures that will reduce the likelihood of having a subsequent loss. The vast array of emotions experienced during the grieving process makes it difficult to systematically and thoughtfully evaluate options to address these important life decisions. Moreover, when the decision involves medical treatment, it is often difficult to obtain the necessary information from medical professionals in a form that is understandable and that will be useful to you. This chapter presents steps for problem solving and decision making in a manner that is appropriate for life decisions such as these. It identifies cognitive and behavioral obstacles that can interfere with problem solving and decision making and describes ways to overcome them, many of which are strategies that have been described earlier in the book.

STEPS OF PROBLEM SOLVING

In this section, I describe the tried-and-true steps to problem solving. These steps may seem rote, boring, or even irrelevant when you are facing decisions as important and meaningful as those associated with a reproductive loss. Nevertheless, I include them as a guide that you may consult when you are overwhelmed and faced with multiple decisions along the way of your reproductive journey.

Problem Definition

Sometimes it helps just to define the problem. I realize that it is pretty clear what the overall problem to be solved is—*have a healthy baby or figure out why I experienced the loss*. However, thinking about problems in such broad terms can be overwhelming, giving you little guidance as to what you should do first. Breaking the problem down into small pieces will give you a better sense of what, specifically, needs to be done. When the pieces have been identified, you will be able to prioritize them. With fertility and reproductive health, much of your prioritization will be based on timing. Certain tasks need to be accomplished before moving onto another task, and the focus of the latter task will be determined, at least in part, from the results of the first task.

Amelia, for example, found that her mind was "running a million miles a minute" in the 3 months after her loss. Although her overall goal was to start trying to become pregnant again as soon as she received clearance to do so, she was strongly encouraged to consult with a physician because until she had experienced her loss, she had been seeing a team of midwives. Thus, the first specific problem that Amelia identified was to identify and make an appointment with an obstetrician. Subsequently, the obstetrician that she chose recommended several courses of action. First, she suggested that Amelia undergo a hysterosalpingogram (HSG) to determine whether there was anything abnormal about her uterus. Second, she anticipated that Amelia would need to go to a compound pharmacy and obtain an injectable progesterone mix at around Week 18 of a subsequent pregnancy to decrease the odds that she would experience another preterm loss. Obviously, the second task needed to be addressed only in the event that she became pregnant again; thus, Amelia recorded this information on a piece of paper to be filed in her "Pregnancy" file and to be consulted at a later time if needed. Next, Amelia moved onto addressing the next tangible and immediate issue of scheduling the HSG.

In contrast, when Jill first started fertility treatment, she continued to be overwhelmed when she broke down "fertility treatment" into smaller pieces. After her initial consultation with her fertility doctor, she was instructed to schedule a number of specific visits, such as a postcoital examination, an HSG, a mammogram, and, for her husband, a semen analysis. All of these visits needed to be scheduled in specific time frames, determined on the basis of where she was in her cycle and the availability of specialty staff in the clinic. Depending on the results of these tests, additional tests and procedures might be needed. Jill had found the paperwork given to her by the fertility clinic to be quite confusing, so she drew her own chart indicating when each test would take place and what, specifically, she and her husband would need to do to meet the demands of the procedure (and, at times, when specifically they needed to complete these activities, such as for the postcoital examination). On a separate sheet of paper, Jill wrote "Next Steps" and described the additional tests and procedures that might need to be conducted, as well as their rationale.

Generation of Alternative Solutions

I view the generation of alternative solutions as a critical stage in problem solving. When you are overwhelmed, it is natural to just want the problem to be over and the decision to be made. However, it often is in your best interest to take some time to brainstorm an array of potential solutions to ensure that you have identified the full pool of possibilities. *Brainstorming* means that you generate as many potential solutions as possible without judging or dismissing them. Refraining from judging or dismissing potential solutions is key; time and again, I find that my clients end up choosing a solution that they otherwise would have dismissed. Other clients find that a combination of solutions often works best, and brainstorming the full array of potential solutions provides a context for the creative combination of solutions.

One important suggestion I have is to be sure to write down all potential solutions. You can use a piece of paper, a white board, or even a notes page on your smartphone or tablet device. The reasoning behind my suggestion is that people can keep only so many bits of information in their working memory. Recording one solution allows you to let it go, at least temporarily, and move on to the brainstorming of other potential solutions without having to go back and monitor so that you ensure that you don't forget the potential solutions that you have already identified.

Amelia applied this step when she was looking for an obstetrician with whom to consult about her recent loss. Living in a major metropolitan area, she had many obstetric practices from which to choose. She identified three main practices, each with different strengths and weaknesses: (a) the department of obstetrics at a prestigious university hospital that was about 40 minutes from her home with no traffic, (b) a small women's health clinic that was only 5 minutes from her home, and (c) the department of obstetrics at a suburban hospital that was 10 to 15 minutes from her home. Within each practice, she printed out the profiles of the obstetricians on staff so that she could learn more about their educational backgrounds and specialty areas. In all, she identified 15 obstetricians from which to choose.

When Jill first started fertility treatment, the generation of alternative solutions was a less central step because she had already committed to a fertility specialist, and the steps for the diagnostic workup were clear to her. She followed her doctor's recommendations and subsequently took a medication to stimulate her follicle production and did four rounds of intrauterine insemination (IUI). Unfortunately, she did not become pregnant after these rounds of IUI, and she proceeded to in vitro fertilization (IVF). After four unsuccessful rounds of IVF, the potential options that Jill identified included the following: (a) proceed with IVF with a donor egg, (b) proceed with IVF with a donor egg and a surrogate, (c) abandon assisted reproductive technology and pursue adoption, (d) abandon assisted reproductive technology and keep trying to get pregnant on her own, or (e) discontinue her effort to have children.

Advantages–Disadvantages Analysis

Like brainstorming, the advantages–disadvantages analysis is another important exercise to record in some form or another, rather than simply completing in your head. It allows you to evaluate each of your potential solutions according to whatever dimensions are important to you. Figure 8.1 is an excerpt from Amelia's advantages–disadvantages analysis of her favorite three obstetricians at the different locations. She identified six important dimensions to consider in choosing an obstetrician: (a) specialty in reproductive loss, (b) distance from home, (c) the quality of the obstetrician's educational background, (d) the quality of the reviews written about the obstetrician, (e) the obstetrician's availability, and (f) the quality of the facility at which the obstetrician worked (e.g., does the facility have state-of-the-art technology?). Notice that Amelia assigned pluses (+) and minuses (–) to each obstetrician for each dimension she considered. A plus was given if the criterion was met, and a minus was given if the

FIGURE 8.1. Amelia's Advantages–Disadvantages Analysis			
	Dr. Smith	Dr. Master	Dr. Lehr
Specialty in reproductive loss	+	–	–
Distance from home	–	+	+
Quality of educational background	+	+ +	+
Quality of reviews	+	+	+ +
Availability	–	+	+
Quality of facility	+ +	+	+

criterion was not met. Amelia assigned two pluses if the obstetrician fared particularly well on a particular dimension.

To start your own advantages–disadvantages analysis, identify the dimensions that are particularly important for you to consider as you evaluate the potential solutions. Then, as best as you can, assign pluses and minuses. If a potential solution fares especially well or especially poorly on a dimension, feel free to assign more than one plus or minus. If you're having trouble assigning a plus or a minus (e.g., you might truly feel neutral about some of the solutions), you can assign a "0," meaning that it is neither an advantage nor a disadvantage.

This is not the only way of doing an advantages–disadvantages analysis. It might be difficult for you to identify a pool of specific dimensions, or you might find that the advantages and disadvantages are quite different depending on the nature of the potential solution, making the pool of specific dimensions unwieldy. This was the case for Jill, who generated five different potential solutions after four rounds of unsuccessful IVF, many of which came with their own unique strengths and challenges. Thus, Jill decided to make a table consisting of three columns—Column 1 listed the different solutions, Column 2 allowed her to record the advantages of each solution, and Column 3 allowed her to record the disadvantages of each solution. Figure 8.2 displays Jill's advantages–disadvantages analysis set up in this manner.

Regardless of whether you choose to conduct an advantages–disadvantages analysis in the manner that Amelia did, in the manner that Jill did, or in a different manner, I strongly encourage you to write it down on paper and carefully consider all angles of all of the solutions. It is easy to decide impulsively on a solution that feels right in your heart, neglecting consideration of some of the practicalities or even the realities of the situation you are facing. The advantages–disadvantages analysis is a tool that allows you to put systematic and productive thought into your decision (without spinning your wheels over and over in a manner that keeps you stuck).

Making a Decision

One way to make a final decision is to examine the number of pluses and minuses for each potential solution. When Amelia did this, she saw that Drs. Masters and Lehr both had six minuses, whereas Dr. Smith had five pluses. She concluded that both Drs. Masters and Lehr were reputable doctors and that it was important that the physician was located relatively close to her home so that she did not spend long hours in traffic. Amelia decided to call both of these doctors' offices and take whichever was the first available appointment. Although she made this firm decision, she still found herself wondering if Dr. Smith would have something more to offer her because he specialized in reproductive loss. She decided to make an appointment with Dr. Smith as well (which was scheduled several months away due to the doctor's lack of availability) to "cover her bases." She reasoned that a consultation with Dr. Smith could yield valuable information with which either Dr. Masters or Dr. Lehr could work. This example illustrates the fact that many solutions involve a combination of the

FIGURE 8.2. Jill's Advantages–Disadvantages Analysis

Potential Solution	Advantages	Disadvantages
IVF—donor egg	High success rate	Would not be biologically related to my child Invasive, time-consuming, and expensive
IVF—donor egg + surrogate	High success rate Would not have to endure a pregnancy	Would not be biologically related to my child Time-consuming and even more expensive than if I would carry the child Not sure how I feel about introducing a surrogate into our lives
Adoption	High success rate Would not have to endure a pregnancy Would be doing something good for a child	Would not be biologically related to my child Time-consuming and expensive Worries about telling the child he or she was adopted, and the biological mother coming back into our lives
Keep trying on own	Would be biologically related to my child No more fertility appointments	Very low success rate Continued stress and uncertainty associated with the threat of not having a child
Decide not to have children	Stress and uncertainty eliminated Could focus on cultivating other areas of my life	Would not have a child

possible solutions that were generated. This often allows for a more thorough approach to problem solving than any one solution alone.

Jill, in contrast, had a more difficult time with her decision-making process. Many of the advantages and disadvantages were based on a balance between cost and probability of success. Moreover, as stated previously, Jill also experienced difficulty estimating how she would feel in the future if she had a child to whom she was not biologically related or did not carry. She knew, however, that giving up the process altogether and not moving forward with parenthood, although indeed associated with some advantages, was not the right solution for her because having a child was important to her. Thus, she narrowed the choices down to IVF using a donor egg or adopting, and she and her husband decided to make one attempt at IVF using a donor egg before pursuing adoption.

At times, you will do a thorough advantages–disadvantages analysis and identify a solution that seems optimal on the basis of the weights of the pluses and minuses. Yet when you go to settle on the final decision, your heart takes you elsewhere, and you choose a solution that is different from the one that the analysis suggested. Angela, for example, had undergone a dangerous ectopic pregnancy that rendered some damage to her fallopian tubes. Her doctor indicated that her chances of conceiving naturally were low and that if she did conceive, there was an elevated likelihood that she would have another ectopic pregnancy. The results of her advantages–disadvantages analysis clearly indicated that she should choose an alternative route to having a child, such as finding a surrogate or adopting, for the sake of her health and safety. However, in her heart, Angela knew that she wanted to try one last time to conceive naturally and carry a child. Thus, she began trying again under the close supervision of her obstetrician.

This example goes to show that you can be systematic in your decision-making process, and you still might ultimately decide on a solution that defies the advantages–disadvantages analysis. That's OK. Fertility decisions are among the most personal and significant decisions you'll make in your life. Only you can choose which direction to take. And you're allowed to change your mind. My strongest recommendation is that you hold off on making major decisions until the acute grief subsides, because it is difficult to concentrate, reason through decisions thoughtfully, and do the research you need to do to be comfortable with your decision. Then, when you make your decision, do so thoughtfully and systematically, even if your ultimate decision involves some risk. The keys are to make the decision in a thoughtful manner and to ensure that the decided-on solution is consistent with your values.

Implementing the Solution

The next step in the problem-solving process is implementing the solution. Some decisions are relatively simple to implement, such as making a telephone call and scheduling an appointment with a physician. Other solutions take some skill, such as the communication skills described in the previous chapter. If the implementation of a solution requires more than one step, I recommend that you carefully walk yourself through that implementation so that you gain some practice before you actually do it. This is called *imaginal rehearsal*, and it increases the likelihood that the implementation of the solution will run smoothly.

Solution implementation can also involve the identification of potential obstacles and ways to overcome those obstacles. Not only does planning ahead for obstacles increase the likelihood that your solution will be successful, it also prepares you so that you are not caught off guard when you encounter them. For example, throughout her fertility treatments, Jill was well aware that there were many possible side effects associated with injectable medications that were used in combination with IVF, and she planned ahead regarding the manner in which she would deal with them if and when they arose. This being said, if you plan ahead too much, you might be plagued by the "what if's" and end up being paralyzed, unable to move forward. Thus, it is important to maintain a healthy balance—objectively identifying potential obstacles and planning for them, but not getting so wrapped up in every possible obstacle that you become overwhelmed, and inertia sits in.

Evaluating the Solution

Many people believe that problem solving is finished after one implements the solution. In actuality, there is an important final step: evaluating the degree to which the solution was effective. Evaluating the effectiveness of a solution gives you important feedback. It's terrific if the solution works out the way you predict. However, in many instances, the solution works only in part. When Amelia attempted to make the appointment at the office that housed both Drs. Masters and Lehr, she was surprised to find that they were not taking new patients despite the fact that her research suggested that they had availability. However, a new physician was joining the practice, and Amelia determined that the new physician had similar educational credentials and experience as Drs. Masters and Lehr. Thus, she decided to make an appointment with the new physician.

It's important to have the realization that a problem might not get solved exactly the way you want it to get solved and that this is OK. It's easy to fall into the trap of all-or-nothing thinking when the solution does not work out, concluding something like "See? Nothing ever works my way." The reality is that life throws curveballs even when the most elegantly designed solution is implemented. Expecting the solution to work out perfectly has the potential to set you up for a great deal of disappointment.

Here is another way to look at a solution that does not entirely achieve its desired outcome: It's a learning opportunity. The experience could allow you to evaluate whether you need to refine aspects of your approach to problem solving or address other skills that are needed to enact the solution. It could help you to refine your expectations and move toward a sense of acceptance over things you cannot control. It could enable you to develop a tolerance for uncertainty, discomfort, and things that do not go as planned. In other words, it is an opportunity for you to make meaning of the experience, just as I hope you will be able to make meaning of your reproductive loss. All of this will help you to stay centered and effective when you face additional life problems in the future.

Putting It All Together

In my experience, I have found that most people find the steps of problem solving to be easy and logical. When I educate people about the steps, the most common response is, "Yeah, yeah. I already know this." However, I have also found that most people, if they are honest with themselves, do not follow these steps systematically; they cut corners, fail to brainstorm the full array of possible solutions, and omit a systematic advantages–disadvantages analysis. Many decisions associated with your reproductive health are just too important and meaningful to omit one or more steps of effective problem solving. For your convenience, I have created a workspace for you to apply these problem-solving steps in Figure 8.3.

COMPLICATIONS IN PROBLEM SOLVING

Some people find that they encounter complications that prevent them from fully embracing the problem-solving approach described in this chapter. If you find yourself too overwhelmed or scattered to implement the problem-solving steps described so far, don't worry.

FIGURE 8.3. Your Personalized Problem-Solving Worksheet

STEP 1: List the problems to be solved, and circle the problem that is of highest priority or that needs to be solved most immediately.

_____   _____

_____   _____

_____   _____

_____   _____

STEP 2: Brainstorm possible solutions to the problem that you have identified.

_____   _____

_____   _____

_____   _____

STEP 3: Conduct an advantages–disadvantage analysis in whatever format makes the most sense to you.

STEP 4: Decide on a solution, and write down why you decided on that solution (or combination of solutions).

(continued)

FIGURE 8.3. Your Personalized Problem-Solving Worksheet (*Continued*)

STEP 5: List the steps to implement the solution, potential obstacles you might encounter, and ways you will overcome those obstacles.

Steps to implement the solution.

_____

_____

_____

_____

Potential Obstacles	Ways to Overcome the Obstacles

STEP 6: Evaluate the solution. What worked, and what did not? What did you learn by implementing the solution?

_____

_____

It might be that you need to work on some other areas of your emotional well-being before you attempt to solve major problems or make major decisions. Decisions regarding reproductive health are tricky because the notion of the biological clock is so ingrained in us. However, even if you accurately perceive that the biological clock is an issue for you, you still have some time to center yourself before making a final decision. In the next sections, I describe some complications that survivors of pregnancy loss might encounter.

Continued Grief

A main message of this book is that everyone is individual in the grieving process—there is no right and wrong. Even if it has been several months since the reproductive loss, you still may feel like you're in a state of acute grief. Although this is entirely OK, I would encourage you to refrain from making major life decisions while you are experiencing acute grief. When you are experiencing acute grief, it is tough to focus and concentrate. Moreover, you might make a hasty decision because you might feel as if a decision cannot wait to be made. Give yourself the time you need to begin healing, and you will be able to address your problems when you are ready to do so.

Negative Problem Orientation

Recall that, in Chapter 6, I defined a *problem orientation* as a cognitive set that one brings to a problem, disagreement, or conflict. In that chapter, I encouraged you to adopt a relationship-focused problem orientation, such that you address disconnect in the partner relationship from the perspective that works best for the relationship, rather than for you as an individual. The concept of the problem orientation has also been incorporated into research that examines helpful and unhelpful ways that people approach problems in their lives.

According to two renowned problem-solving researchers, Tom D'Zurilla and Art Nezu, a *negative problem orientation* is an unhelpful way of viewing problems that interferes with the execution of problem solving. It is not a deficit in actual problem-solving skills. Rather, it is a cognitive style characterized by the tendencies to (a) view problems as bad, rather than challenging; (b) view problems as unsolvable, rather than solvable; (c) believe that one does not have the ability to solve problems; (d) fail to accept that problems are a part of life; and (e) recognize that problem solving

195

takes time and effort. I realize that now probably won't seem like the time to work systematically toward modifying a negative problem orientation. However, if you at least have insight into what it is, the distress that you are experiencing when you think about addressing your reproductive problems will be understandable and explainable. Once you have made some decisions about your reproductive future and feel as though you are out of the crisis associated with your reproductive loss, you might want to work on modifying a negative problem orientation. It will help you to weather problems that you encounter in all kinds of areas of your life. In other words, investing the time to create a more helpful problem orientation will be associated with benefits for years to come.

If you do choose to work on a negative problem orientation right now, here are some things to consider. Do you view problems as bad? If so, take some time to think objectively about your past and identify other instances in which you encountered problems in your life. Write them down on a sheet of paper in one column. Now, in the other column, write down what the outcome of the problem was. Circle the outcomes that turned out to be at least somewhat positive. More often than not, we view problems as bad because of the uncertainty associated with them. But in reality, there are many, many instances when the problem ultimately gets resolved, even if it was in a manner different from what was expected. The items on this list will serve as important pieces of evidence against the notion that problems are bad and that things do not work out when problems occur. Think about the number of times you hear people saying that they would not be where they are today had they not encountered a problem that prompted them to take their lives in a different direction. What I often say to my clients who struggle with reproductive loss and trauma is to think of how sweet the "victory" will be if and when they finally have a child, given the struggles they have endured. These clients agree that there is no question that they will savor moments with their child and that their child will be especially loved in light of their reproductive circumstances.

Do you view problems as unsolvable? There is likely to be a subset of readers who have been given the devastating news that they will not be able to bear children. There is no question that this news is heartbreaking and takes much time to process and accept. However, keep in mind that even this is a situation in which the problem of having children can be solvable if one thinks outside the box and broadens one's definition of what it means to have children (e.g., through surrogacy, adoption). Thus, a redefinition of the problem can help you move from a truly solvable situation to a situation in which creative solutions exist.

Do you believe that you do not have the ability to solve problems, such that you get overwhelmed too easily? If so, I would encourage you to do two things. First, practice the problem-solving steps described earlier in this chapter with small problems, and work toward solving larger ones. It's almost the same idea as the hierarchy described in Chapter 7—begin with tasks that are of mild to moderate levels of difficulty and move toward tasks that are of great difficulty. Doing this will allow you to have successful experiences that will serve as pieces of evidence that contradict the idea that you are unable to solve problems. Second, think back to the times when you solved problems in the past, and write them down on a sheet of paper. This listing will serve as a reminder of the times when you were successful in solving problems, which provides evidence that is contrary to the idea that you do not have the ability to do so. When you think back to the times when you successfully solved problems, you might remember what actions you took, which could have relevance to solving a current problem.

Notice that this is the second time I have encouraged you to write a list of previous problems: The first time I asked you to list problems for which the ultimate outcome was OK or even favorable;

this time I asked you to list problems that you solved successfully. It is likely that there is a great deal of overlap between these lists. Although the idea of writing a list like these might seem artificial, I view the information on this list as a crucial reminder that can soften a negative problem orientation. In fact, research shows that when people feel sad and down, they tend to have difficulty remembering specific positive experiences in their past, which in turn affects their ability to solve current problems because they are unable to access in memory previous instances in which they solved problems successfully. This tendency is called an *overgeneral memory style*. By compiling one or both of these lists, you will circumvent the overgeneral memory style, be reminded of reasons you can have confidence in your problem-solving ability, and recall, specifically, previous ways you solved problems that might have relevance to your current life problems.

WHEN THE SOLUTION DOESN'T WORK: WHAT'S NEXT?

In an ideal world, the solution you implement will address your problem. However, in reality, you will encounter instances in which the solution that you have enacted does not work or perhaps works to some degree, but not fully. In these cases, it is important not to fall into the all-or-nothing thinking trap, such that you believe you have failed or that things will never work out, if the solution you have implemented does not achieve its desired effect. It may be that you need to try again. It may be that it would behoove you to have a Plan B prepared if Plan A does not work out. It may be that you would benefit from coming to a sense of acceptance of the parts of the problem that are not within your control or that will not work out to your liking.

Most people who have experienced a reproductive loss are very invested in finding a solution to their problems and have often devoted more of their time, energy, and emotional resources to solving this problem than in solving any other problem in their lives. It can be devastating when it does not work out as you had planned. Use the tools described throughout this book to take care of yourself and find meaning in your struggle. Once you have grieved the loss of your reproductive story, you will find ways to redefine your goals and live according to your values, even if you do so in a manner than is much different from what you had envisioned for yourself.

PROBLEM SOLVING IN THE FACE OF UNCERTAINTY

It's human nature to experience anxiety and trepidation when you are faced with a situation that you view as uncontrollable and unpredictable. It is true that there are many, many aspects of fertility and reproductive health that are uncontrollable and unpredictable. Moreover, there are many aspects of fertility and reproductive health that are overwhelming and confusing. Not only will you likely be sorting through lots of information and materials that are given to you by health care professionals as well as those obtained through your own research, you will also likely find that some of the information contradicts other information. It's not difficult to see how these circumstances, coupled with the intense emotions surrounding a reproductive loss, can result in a sense of paralysis, helplessness, powerlessness, and hopelessness. If this has been your experience, you are not alone.

The systematic application of the problem-solving and decision-making skills described in this chapter provides one way for you to reclaim a small bit of control and predictability. By using these skills, you will ensure that you (a) will not miss a possible and viable solution that you otherwise would have dismissed or overlooked; (b) thoroughly review your options to arrive at a reasoned decision, rather than one that is impulsive or based entirely on emotions; (c) have reasonable expectations for the likelihood of success; (d) identify obstacles that have the potential to interfere with implementing a solution and ways to overcome those obstacles; and (e) develop backup plans or alternatives if your solutions do not achieve their desired effects. The hardest part of all of this, however, is that none of this guarantees the outcome that you want. Moreover, it can be months, or even years, before you know the final outcome, and the wait can be excruciating. In the next chapter, I describe some strategies for achieving acceptance of the uncertainty surrounding fertility as well as surrounding outcomes that are undesired. I encourage readers to use these acceptance strategies hand-in-hand with the problem-solving and decision-making tools described in this chapter.

CHAPTER 9

STAYING MINDFUL AND ACHIEVING ACCEPTANCE

If you're reading this book, it's likely that you have experienced a reproductive loss or trauma that you so desperately did not want to happen and that you would not wish even on your worst enemy. It's possible that you have lived through your worst or most dreaded fear. As has been discussed in many instances in this book, it's easy to ruminate over how unfair life is, to become angry and bitter, and to be petrified about what the future holds. It's easy to fight back against your reality, suffering tremendously as you struggle against acceptance over what has happened.

A wise mentor once told me that 90% of one's experience of pain, whether it be physical or emotional, is actually the suffering. Think of what happens when you wake up in the middle of the night to go to the bathroom and you trip on something and stub your toe. There is the physical sensation of pain that emanates through your toes and foot, perhaps even up your lower leg. But more often than not, there is a secondary reaction: "My gosh, I am so clumsy, I can't believe I did that, or My partner is so inconsiderate! How could she leave her shoes out in the open, right where I could trip on them?" This secondary reaction is what I regard as the *suffering*, or the *struggle*. It is this suffering reaction to the pain that intensifies the experience of the pain, as well as one's ability to accept the pain and recover. In this chapter, I consider ways to overcome this secondary struggle reaction and, in doing so, help you to form a new relationship with the emotional pain associated with your reproductive loss. It is my hope that you will, after reading this chapter, be able to identify instances in which rumination over the past or worry about the future (i.e., the suffering or struggle) has taken away from a present-focused approach to living, acquire strategies to let go of the struggle in your daily life, contemplate acceptance of the loss, and understand the manner in which these strategies work and promote healing.

MINDFULNESS

Mindfulness is a practice that is increasingly being incorporated into mainstream psychology as a way to reduce the struggle against physical and emotional pain. Although mindfulness was originally practiced by Zen Buddhists thousands of years ago, mindfulness practice is now being incorporated in a secular manner into medicine, psychotherapy, and stress reduction programs. One person who played an instrumental role in bringing mindfulness to modern medicine is Jon Kabat-Zinn, who is Professor Emeritus of the University of Massachusetts School of Medicine and author of many popular books on mindfulness. In his renowned book *Wherever You Go, There You Are* (1994), Kabat-Zinn defined mindfulness as "paying attention in a particular way: on purpose, in the present moment, and nonjudgmentally" (p. 4). The implementation of these three components is central to living a valued life. *Paying attention on purpose* means that one is thoughtfully focused on one thing, rather than checking out or being distracted by doing several things at once. *Being in the present moment* means that one is focused on the here and now, rather than ruminating about the past or worrying about the future. And *nonjudgmentally* means that one is accepting the moment as it is, rather than worrying about when it will end, hoping it will end, wishing it away, or lamenting how bad the moment is. In other words, being in the present moment on purpose and nonjudgmentally means that one is letting go of the struggle against whatever pain he or she is experiencing.

On the previous page, I mentioned that you can achieve a new relationship with your pain. Let me elaborate on that notion. When a person is experiencing physical or emotional pain, the struggle against it occurs in the form of judgments, such as judgments about how awful it is, judgments about how it isn't fair, and judgments about how it will negatively affect one's life. With all of these judgments, it's not surprising that we're quite fearful of experiencing pain, we experience dread when we are faced with pain, and we go to great lengths to avoid it. In other words, pain is daunting. But when you adopt a nonjudgmental mindful stance to understand pain, you are experiencing it is for what it is, not for what it means about you or about your life. You are observing the actual sensations rather than their implications. Mindfulness masters, such as Jon Kabat-Zinn, encourage practitioners of mindfulness to even adopt a curious stance as they observe the sensations associated with their pain. When you adopt such a stance, the pain will no longer seem as threatening. And although the pain will still be there, by letting go of the associated judgment and struggle, you will reduce the secondary emotional distress associated with the pain.

I believe that everyone could benefit from mindfulness training. It helps people stop to smell the roses when there are roses to be smelled, which enhances quality of life and buffers against depression. But it also allows people to experience and endure the times when there are no roses, during times of stress, challenge, and loss. Mindfulness is especially relevant to reproductive loss, given the rumination about the past and excessive worrying about the future in which people who have experienced reproductive loss often engage that takes them out of the present moment and potentially exacerbates their emotional disturbance. In this section, I present some techniques that you can use to begin to acquire skill in mindfulness, and I describe how they can serve as a vehicle for healing and can be implemented in your daily life. I cannot take credit for any of the exercises described in this section; they are part of standard mindfulness programs that have been described in countless books and websites, especially mindfulness-based cognitive therapy (MBCT) developed by Zindel Segal, John Teasdale, and Mark Williams. In the appendix of this book, I list some of these resources that you can consult for more information.

Mindfulness Exercises

When people first embark on mindfulness practice, their first reaction is, "easier said than done!" I agree that it is difficult to switch into a mindful way of being without systematic and graduated practice. The following exercises are designed to give you a framework for practicing mindfulness in small doses, with the idea that you will build up skill over time and eventually be able to adopt a mindful approach to living your life even when you are not following a prescribed exercise.

MINDFUL EATING. A standard introduction to mindfulness and many mindfulness programs, such as MBCT, is something called the *raisin exercise*. If I were seeing you in my practice in person, I would give you a raisin and ask you to examine it as if you were an alien, as if you have never seen anything like it before. In fact, I wouldn't even refer to it as a "raisin"; instead, I would refer to it as an "object" so that you would not have any preconceived notions (i.e., judgments) about what a raisin entails. I would lead you through a sequence of rolling the object around in your hand, examining its peaks and valleys, meditating on the manner in which the light hits different parts of the object, bringing the object outside of the nose and inhaling its aroma, bringing the object outside of the mouth and noticing the manner in which the mouth knows that there is food outside of it, rolling the object around the tongue, taking a bite and noticing the taste of both the inside and the outside of the object, swallowing the object, and reflecting on the fact that you are now exactly one raisin heavier.

It might seem very different from the manner in which you would typically eat a raisin. However, consider the type of reaction I typically get from my clients after they have participated in this activity: "Wow, I never knew there was so much going on with raisins. When I eat them, I usually shovel them in my mouth mindlessly, not paying attention to how it looks, feels, smells, and tastes." Mindfully eating the raisin introduced a whole new eating experience, such that my clients could absorb and appreciate the intricacies of the raisin, which, to that point, had usually gone unnoticed.

This sort of exercise helps people to recognize when they are operating on *automatic pilot*, or when they are in a mode in which they are going through the motions of life and not present with the rich intricacies that life has to offer. Living in this manner has the potential to deprive us of the small pleasures that can be derived from everyday experience. However, it also plays a role in your emotional distress. When you are living in automatic pilot mode, you might not notice the subtle signs or indicators that emotional distress is coming on, when you can take a step back, center yourself, and do something skillful to manage it. Thus, living mindfully helps you to manage emotional distress because you detect it sooner than you would if you are living in automatic pilot mode, and you will be able to implement the tools and skills described in this book to do something about it.

There is no doubt that it takes practice to live in a mindful mode, rather than in automatic pilot mode. However, mindful eating is one way for you to practice slowing down and moving out of automatic pilot mode to truly engage the senses as you eat. You might try it with a single food item, such as a raisin, nut, or piece of candy. Alternatively, you might try it as you are eating a dish that has many ingredients, such as a salad. I have had other clients mindfully engage the senses as they were cooking a meal and tasting the fruits of their work. In addition to learning how to step out of automatic pilot mode, you might even obtain a small sense of joy or pleasure from the food you are eating, which is yet another antidote against sadness and depression.

One word of caution, though: Do not go into this exercise *expecting* to obtain a sense of joy or pleasure. Those expectations mask themselves as another form of judgment, and they may set you up to be disappointed. The goal of mindfulness is not exactly to feel better, or calm down, or achieve some sort of other positive outcome. If that happens, terrific. But it might not happen, and the idea is that you will be just as mindful during those times as you are when the exercise helps you to feel better. The goal of mindfulness, then, is to fully experience the moment as it is, whatever it is.

MINDFULNESS OF EVERYDAY ACTIVITIES. Another way to practice stepping out of automatic pilot mode is to practice mindfulness during an everyday activity that you usually do in a thoughtless, automatic manner. The purpose of this exercise is the same as mindful eating—it shows you just how much you live your life in automatic pilot mode and the richness of your experience if you engage in the activity from a more mindful stance. It allows you to connect to the present moment in a new way.

My favorite everyday activity to which you can apply mindfulness is brushing your teeth. The most typical times of the day in which people brush their teeth—first thing in the morning and right before bed—are also the most typical times in which we are in automatic pilot mode, partially zoning out in a fog of tiredness. On first glance, it might not seem that there is much to brushing your teeth. However, after practicing mindful toothbrushing, you might feel differently. You might notice the aroma of the toothpaste. You might focus on the texture of the toothpaste and the feel of the toothbrush in different parts of your mouth, such as the teeth, gums, and tongue. You might compare and contrast the temperature of the toothpaste stored at room temperature and the cold water you are using to rinse. You might notice the movement of the bristles of your toothbrush. In other words, there is much more to toothbrushing than meets the eye, and doing it mindfully has the potential to remind you of the rich variations of this experience.

BODY SCAN. The *body scan* is a third exercise that helps people to step out of automatic pilot. To practice the body scan, lie flat or in a reclining position, and systematically direct your attention to various muscle groups in turn. Although this might sound a lot like muscle relaxation, described in Chapter 2, there are some important differences. First, this exercise does not require you to tense and relax the various muscle groups as you do in muscle relaxation; the idea, instead, is for you just to notice what is happening in the muscle groups. It allows you to notice tension or other sensations associated with various emotional experiences. Some people find that the body scan can be somewhat uncomfortable when they notice tension in various parts of the body. If this describes you, I would encourage you to "breathe into" and "breathe out of" those muscle groups, infusing the centeredness of your breath into those areas of tension. After you have practiced the exercise, see if you can expand your focus of attention to the body as a whole, as one unit that breathes in and breathes out in synchronicity.

How do mindfulness exercises like mindful eating, mindful practice of everyday activities, and the body scan help a person work through a devastating reproductive loss? They provide valuable lessons on just how often you are operating in automatic pilot mode, as well as what you are missing when you operate in automatic pilot mode. Right now, you might feel a sense of numbness, as though you are just going through the motions of life. Practicing mindfulness to step out of automatic pilot mode can help you, then, to reengage in a more meaningful way with your life.

And, as stated earlier, you will notice subtle signs of emotional distress sooner than you otherwise might have. This occurred for Kristin, who seemed to experience an exacerbation of her emotional distress around the sixth day of each month, the date at which she lost her baby. Although she understood the pattern, she tried to avoid the emotional pain at all costs, multitasking in an unmindful manner so that she could push it away. However, without fail, it would return with a vengeance and would overtake her, often to the point at which she would have to call in sick to work. After practicing mindfulness and learning to step out of automatic pilot, Kristin recognized that the first sign that her emotional distress was coming on was tension in her neck and upper shoulders. Thus, she was more mindful of these sensations, and when she detected them, she was able to implement a self-care plan to lessen the blow of the pain associated with the reminder of her loss. She did not eliminate her emotional pain, but she was able to take skillful action to manage it in a healthy, adaptive manner.

MINDFULNESS OF THE BREATH. *Mindfulness of the breath* is perhaps the single most important mindfulness exercise to take away from this chapter. Some people find mindfulness of the breath more challenging than the mindful practice of a particular activity. Nevertheless, I view it as central to mindfulness practice because you always have your breath with you, and you can use it to practice mindfulness in any circumstance without having to find a raisin, a toothbrush and sink, and so on.

Quite simply, mindfulness of the breath involves a following of the breath through each inbreath and each outbreath. You don't have to change your breathing in any way; you just pay attention to the air going into your nose or mouth and to the air going out of your nose or mouth. You can pay attention to your muscles as you breathe, such as your diaphragm that moves up and down as you breathe in and out. You can notice the manner in which your belly expands as you breathe in and out. You can observe the sensations of your breath in your nose or your mouth. Many people who are acquiring skill in mindfulness practice mindful breathing for approximately 10 minutes every day. In the appendix, I have listed resources where you can gain access to audio versions of mindfulness exercises, all of which have a version of mindfulness of the breath, so that you can listen to a soothing voice leading you through it.

After you have had practice with mindfulness of the breath, you can condense it into what is called the *3-minute breathing space* in MBCT. The 3-minute breathing space prescribes three steps to follow in harnessing the power of the breath in any one moment: (a) awareness of one's experience in the present moment, (b) gathering of one's attention to the process of breathing, and (c) expanding one's awareness to include a sense of the body as a whole. I have had many clients who claim that the 3-minute breathing space is an excellent tool for remaining centered and balanced, such as when they are sorting through a barrage of e-mails, all of which are demanding immediate action. I believe that mindfulness of the breath is a particularly important tool for people who have experienced reproductive loss because it provides a way to stay centered in a sea of overwhelming emotions.

MINDFUL PHYSICAL ACTIVITY. Some people find that they gravitate toward mindfulness exercises that involve some sort of physical activity. For example, mindful walking allows you to focus on each of your steps and the movement of lifting one leg and setting down the other. People often find that the rhythmic movement helps them to coordinate their steps with their breath and facilitate a sense of mindfulness. Marsha Linehan, a renowned researcher who has incorporated mindfulness into her unique cognitive behavioral treatment package called dialectical behavioral therapy, encourages practitioners of mindfulness to cultivate, with each step, an awareness of their connection to the earth. In addition, yoga is an activity that shares many principles with mindfulness, such as a present focus and reliance on the breath. You can do yoga in your home, or you can go out and take a class. One benefit of taking a class is that not only will you have access to an expert who can help you to hone your mindfulness and yoga skills, it also facilitates active engagement with one's life and social connection, which have been discussed in previous chapters as having important antidepressant effects. Other types of physical activities that lend themselves to mindfulness include stretching, swimming, and rowing.

MINDFUL ABSORPTION OF NATURE. As has been implied in this discussion so far, mindfulness is particularly engaging when one can involve several of the senses—touch, smell, sight, hearing, and taste. I encourage my clients to practice mindfulness when they are surrounded by nature and to fully engage the senses. If it is autumn, mindfully take in the aroma of leaves on the ground, feel the cool air against your cheek, and visually take in the radiant fall colors. If it is winter, mindfully take in the aroma of pine trees; feel the snowflakes land on your face; savor the warmth of your winter coat, gloves, scarf, and hat; and visually take in the white landscape. If it is spring, mindfully take in the aroma of freshly cut grass or lilacs, pay attention to what it feels like to have the sun on your face after so many months without it, and visually take in the vivid greens, pinks, purples, and yellows. If you live in the mountains or near the beach, don't let a day go by in which you don't take a moment to savor your surroundings. Even if you live in an urban area, take a walk to a park, notice the flowers and trees that are planted along the roadways, or even savor your city's own version of "nature" (e.g., lights, holiday decorations, fancy architecture).

The point is that your surroundings allow you to step out of automatic pilot and engage your senses. This will help you to feel alive, and it might even allow you a sense of soothing. In addition, you might notice some of the little joys or pleasures that you have overlooked in the past, such as the sweet sound of the birds singing or the intricate pattern of the clouds in the sky. Mindful awareness of such small beauties is another thing that I believe contributes to a valued life.

MINDFUL EXPERIENCING OF EMOTIONS. After you have had some practice with the mindfulness activities described to this point, try to turn your attention to the mindful awareness of your emotional experiences themselves. This means that you will sit with your emotions, whatever they are, happy, painful, or neutral, without judging them. Practicing mindfulness of your emotional experiences will help you to accept the emotions that you are experiencing in any one moment, rather than pushing them away. You may find that you experience thoughts that accompany your emotional experiences, and if these emotional experiences are decidedly negative, it's possible that some of these thoughts might even be disturbing to you. Here, I will remind you of a theme that is emphasized in MBCT: Thoughts are just thoughts; they are just neural activities going on in your brain; thoughts are not facts. These thoughts and emotions do not have to hold power over you; they are simply your experience in the moment and do not have to determine your experience in the next moment.

Try viewing your emotions and thoughts as clouds that are passing by in the sky, such that the cloud enters your head on one side, gently passes through, and leaves out the other side. Or as a movie that goes by, frame-by-frame, such that there is momentary focus on one frame before the next frame is projected onto the screen. I like to view each moment in life as being on a pendulum. Think about the nature of a pendulum—it never stops moving, even if it is relatively centered in the middle and only makes small movements. So, if your pendulum is way off to the right side or the left side after a tragic event such as a reproductive loss, you can have faith that it will not stay in that place forever and will eventually settle back into the middle.

Mindful observation of emotions is perhaps one of the most difficult mindfulness exercises to do, especially when you are experiencing pain, despair, and distress. However, as was described in Chapter 2, the alternative—to push away or otherwise suppress the thoughts—has been shown not to be effective. By accepting your emotional state in any one moment, you are letting go of the struggle against your emotional pain and forming a new relationship with your emotional pain, which should help these emotional experiences to seem less threatening and less daunting.

APPLICATIONS TO THE PERINATAL EXPERIENCES. There are many ways that you can apply mindfulness as you go through your reproductive journey. For example, when she was going for fertility treatment, Karen noticed that the ceiling of the examination rooms had some panels that were painted to look like the sky. As she was going through sometimes-invasive procedures, she paid close attention to these ceiling panels and absorbed the beautiful cloud designs and the radiant blue. Even if you are in examination rooms that do not lend themselves to such visual stimulation, you can nevertheless practice mindfulness of the breath during your procedures. If you experience pain during procedures, you can even breathe into those areas, like you did when you practiced breathing into the tense muscle groups during the body scan.

If you are trying to get pregnant again, it is more than understandable that you feel consumed by the practicalities, such as predicting your ovulation and charting your temperature. When couples are struggling to get pregnant, they often have the sense that the fun and intimacy have been taken out of sexual intercourse, believing that it feels mechanical and it is far from emerging spontaneously. If this description fits you, I would encourage you to apply a mindful attitude to sex with your partner. Notice and savor the feelings of arousal and chemistry between the two of you. If you notice negative emotional experiences such as worry about whether you will become pregnant, just register them as passing internal experiences and know that the next moment might very well be different. My prediction is that the application of mindfulness to sexual intercourse will facilitate a sense of closeness and connection with your partner, which will be another asset that will help you endure this difficult time in your life.

If you get pregnant again, you will likely experience a great deal of anxiety over whether you will experience another loss and whether the baby will be OK. Again, notice these worries and thoughts as internal experiences and remember the pendulum—that the next moment need not be determined by the present moment. Your worries are just thoughts, not facts that will determine or guarantee the outcome of your pregnancy. Many people who have experienced reproductive loss say that they have difficulty enjoying the pregnancy experience and maintain a guarded, detached stance so that they are not devastated if they experience another loss. Of course, this is understandable. However, you might deprive yourself of the opportunity to savor the little joys that help get women through pregnancy. Be mindful of instances of when you feel your baby kick. Or when you hear your baby's heartbeat during your checkups.

Obstacles You Might Encounter

Mindfulness is not a skill that can be cultivated overnight. In fact, many people find mindfulness to be quite frustrating when they first attempt it. In this section, I describe obstacles you might encounter and ways to overcome those obstacles.

My mind races too much to focus on any one thing. This is perhaps the single most common comment I hear from people who are learning mindfulness. Keep this point in mind: It is absolutely natural for minds to wander. It's what minds do. If you have the expectation that you are going to sustain focused attention on one thing for several minutes, you will likely set yourself up for disappointment. Instead, apply a sense of gentle curiosity to the direction in which your mind went. Briefly note whatever it was that captured your mind's attention, and gently bring your attention back to the mindfulness exercise at hand. Know that you are going to move through this process over and over, such that you'll be focused on a mindfulness exercise, that you'll notice that your mind has wandered, that you'll gently notice to where your mind went, and that you'll gently bring your mind back to the mindfulness exercise at hand. In this way, you can view mindfulness as much more of a process than it is as an outcome. Even if you find that your mind has wandered over and over and over, by gently bringing it back to the task at hand, you are practicing mindfulness.

I didn't feel any better. If this is your reaction, remember that the purpose of mindfulness is not necessarily to feel better. You may feel better in some instances, and you may not feel any better in other instances. Rather, the purpose of mindfulness is to fully experience *what is* in the present moment, breathing it in, knowing that they next moment may or may not be different.

I didn't do it right; I must have failed. When they are first learning mindfulness, many people conclude that they are not doing it correctly when their mind wanders, when they do not feel better, or when they experience some sort of enhanced discomfort. I tend not to use the words *right* or *wrong* when I am practicing mindfulness on my own or when I am working with clients to acquire skill in mindfulness, as these terms imply judgment when we are working toward taking a nonjudgmental stance. Remember that mindfulness is more of a process than an outcome. The simple fact that you are challenging yourself to engage in mindfulness practice means that you have not failed.

Therapists who are trained in MBCT often work with clients to map the "territory" of their previous episodes of emotional distress. Often, this territory comprises negative thoughts about oneself, and it is thought that by stepping out of automatic pilot and recognizing times in your life when these thoughts arise quickly and automatically, you will be able to catch a subtle indicator that another episode of emotional distress is percolating, and you can do something skillful to address it. Thus, if you are berating yourself for doing mindfulness wrong or even labeling yourself as a failure, consider the possibility that this judgment may be part of your territory of emotional distress and is actually a signal to use the skills and tools described in this book to address it before it overtakes you.

Many mindfulness experts encourage clients to assume a stance of self-compassion when engaging in mindfulness exercises. Bring a sense of gentle kindness to yourself, regardless of what your experience is in the moment. Know that you have gone through an unspeakable tragedy and that you are doing the best that you can. Remind yourself that you would likely be supportive and compassionate toward a friend or family member who went through an experience like you did and that you deserve the same kindness.

Mindfulness: Caveat

You might recall that I described the symptoms of depression in Chapter 1. The criteria for major depression, a diagnosis of depression that often requires treatment from a mental health professional, are as follows: (a) depressed mood more of the time than not, (b) loss of interest and enjoyment in activities, (c) appetite disturbance or weight loss or gain, (d) sleep disturbance, (e) psychomotor disturbance (i.e., either being fidgety and agitated or moving much more slowly than normal), (f) fatigue, (g) a sense of worthlessness or excessive guilt, (h) difficulty concentrating or indecisiveness, and (i) suicidal thoughts or behaviors. A person meets criteria for major depression when she acknowledges at least five of these criteria, one of which must be either criterion (a) or criterion (b). Of course, it is important for a trained mental health professional to confirm the diagnosis because they consider other factors such as duration of the symptoms, severity of the symptoms, whether the symptoms can be accounted for by other factors, and the degree to which they cause life interference and emotional distress.

I have included discussion of this diagnosis here because experts believe that mindfulness might not be a good match for people who are in the throes of major depression. MBCT, the mindfulness approach to which I've referred throughout the chapter, was developed as a program to prevent relapse and recurrence of depressive symptoms and to be delivered to people who are well into their recovery from depression. There is no question that you might meet these criteria soon after your reproductive loss. However, if they persist for several months, you should consider consulting a mental health professional who can determine whether you indeed meet criteria for major depression. If this is the case, talk with the mental health professional about receiving treatments that have proven efficacy in the treatment of major depression (e.g., cognitive behavioral therapy, which incorporates many of the strategies described in previous chapters of this volume; antidepressant medication). Once the acute symptoms have subsided, you can begin to practice mindfulness meditation.

ACCEPTANCE

Mindfulness is often used in the service of achieving a sense of acceptance. Acceptance of pregnancy loss, unsuccessful fertility treatments, the realization that you might be unable to have biologically related children, the realization that you might have fewer children than you wanted, and so on might seem impossible to achieve because these types of reproductive loss represent the most profound disappointment that you have ever experienced. On the surface, acceptance might feel like giving up or resignation. However, this does not have to be the case. Acceptance can be a decision made from a place of empowerment in which you let go of the struggle against what is; embrace the present moment, whatever that may be; and orient yourself toward living a valued life, even if you have to spend some time redefining the valued life for which you are striving. In other words, you are *choosing* a path of acceptance.

Marsha Linehan, the developer of dialectical behavior therapy, promoted a powerful heuristic for thinking about acceptance by distinguishing *willfulness from willingness. Taking a willful stance* means that you are struggling against the reality of your situation. It might take the form of inaction when action is needed. It might take the form of doing something different from the effective action called for in the moment, even if you have the "right" to take the action that you are taking. It might take the form of trying to fix the situation at all costs. Or it might take the form of refusing to tolerate the distress that you are experiencing in the present moment. I view willfulness as the equivalent of trying to pound a square peg into a round hold.

A *willing stance*, in contrast, is a stance that is inviting. It is doing what is effective in the moment, even if what is happening in that moment is not fair or feels awful, or even if you would rather turn away and hide. It is taking action that is according to your values and the person who you want to be. It is allowing yourself to be connected with the present experience—with your emotion, with your breath, with the person with whom you are talking. The image that comes to my mind when I am thinking about willingness is that of a babbling brook. One cannot stop the brook from babbling. The water flows in a certain direction. The bubbles that arise are continuous. There is a certain peace and tranquility associated with the babbling brook. I often encourage my clients to develop their own image or symbol of willingness. When they are faced with stress, adversity, or a moment of challenge, I encourage them to adopt a decision rule as they decide how to response: "Is my response one of willfulness, or is my response one of willingness, such that I am doing what is effective and embracing, rather than resisting what is?"

I also think of a metaphor developed by my colleague Karen Kleiman, who directs the Postpartum Stress Center in the Philadelphia suburbs and who has authored many books about perinatal depression and anxiety. The metaphor speaks to the effectiveness of gripping tightly (i.e., willfulness) versus letting go (i.e., willingness). Imagine that you are in the midst of a water balloon fight and that you have snagged the last remaining balloon. You want to save the balloon so that you can throw it at just the right moment and win the fight. However, the longer you hold it, the more likely it is that you will drop it, and it will break. What can you do? Many people have the tendency to keep a tight hold on something that they do not want to drop. What happens, though, when you grip a water balloon tightly? It will probably burst or jump out of your hand and burst on the ground. The more effective action, then, is to let go of your grip and let the water balloon balance on your open palm. It may sound counterintuitive, but doing this makes it more likely that the balloon will remain intact and that you will have it when you need it.

Now might be the time to open up your palm and let your water balloon rest in your hand, rather than gripping it tightly. This does not mean that you are resigning yourself to dropping the balloon or losing the water balloon fight altogether. You are doing what's effective, adopting a stance of willingness, even if in the short term it appears that you are taking yourself further away from your goal. With that loosening of your grip will come clarity, a greater sense of peacefulness, and grace and dignity on which you can rely as you navigate your journey.

COMMITMENT TO A LIFELONG MINDFULNESS AND ACCEPTANCE PRACTICE

Although I have described several exercises and heuristics in this chapter to help you practice mindfulness and acceptance, it is most helpful to view mindfulness and acceptance as lifelong ways of being, rather than as discrete activities that you work into your busy schedule. The more you practice these exercises and make decisions according to these heuristics and concepts, the more you will be able approach many, if not all, activities in your life from a mindful, accepting stance. In other words, the more you practice, the more you will live your life in a mindful and accepting manner. I operate under the assumptions that living a mindful, accepting life will improve your life's quality, increase the likelihood that you live according to your values, and help you to let go of the struggle with future stressors and challenges that come your way, allowing you to handle stressors, challenges, and disappointments with the utmost grace and dignity.

How can you commit to living a life characterized by mindfulness and acceptance? Here are a few suggestions:

- Take a class or a series of classes on mindfulness. Many hospitals and medical centers offer classes on mindfulness-based stress reduction, the type of mindfulness that was developed by the expert referenced earlier in this chapter, Jon Kabat-Zinn. You can find these classes by doing an Internet search for *mindfulness-based stress reduction* and the name of your location (or the name of the nearest largest city).
- If you are currently in psychotherapy or think psychotherapy could be beneficial, inquire as to whether the therapist has training in mindfulness-based stress reduction or MBCT. Many certified cognitive behavioral therapists (see http://www.academyofct.org) are able to provide mindfulness training.
- Commit to 10 to 20 minutes of mindfulness practice each day. Using the resources listed in the appendix, you can listen to various audio tracks that lead you through mindfulness exercises. Or you can engage in whatever type of intentional mindfulness practice you would like—mindful eating, mindful walking, mindful yoga, and so on.
- Commit to responding to stress or adversity from a mindful response, rather than one that is reactive, impulsive, or alarmist. Remember that mindfulness allows you to center yourself, connecting with your breath and your emotional experiences, which in turn allows you to take skillful action. Skillful action might include any of the other strategies and tools described in this book, including self-care, behavioral activation, thought modification, problem solving, and effective communication. With my own clients, I refer to this as the "one–two punch,"

such that when faced with stress or adversity, you first take a few moments to focus your attention on the breath, expand your awareness to your body as a whole, and then, when you are centered, use the tried-and-true cognitive and behavioral strategies to take care of yourself, manage emotional distress, solve the problem, and maintain a stance of acceptance.

- Continue reading about mindfulness and acceptance. There are numerous mindfulness resources available to the general public. I highly recommend works written by Jon Kabat-Zinn, Mark Williams, and Thich Nhat Hanh, although these are but three of many, many renowned authors who are committed to bringing mindfulness to mainstream culture. Although many concepts are similar across these books, each book includes its own unique set of mindfulness practices; metaphors for understanding and appreciating mindfulness, acceptance, and willingness; and insights into mindfulness and acceptance that may resonate with you. Examples of these books can be found in the appendix.

Just like healing from a reproductive loss, mindfulness and acceptance are journeys, rather than states that you can achieve overnight. However, much of the benefit you will obtain will come from the process of your journey, rather than any one outcome that you will achieve. Investment in mindfulness and acceptance now will give you a lifetime's worth of skill and wisdom that will be available to you as you face whatever you find on your path.

CHAPTER 10

CREATING A NEW NORMAL
AND FINDING MEANING

As I have stated on many occasions throughout this book, it is a misnomer to state that one simply "gets over" a reproductive loss. This is not to be overly pessimistic. People indeed successfully work through the grief, focus on life goals, and achieve happiness, quality of life, and life satisfaction. It's just that the experience is never forgotten, and most people are transformed in some way after such a profound experience. One key to achieving these positive outcomes is to create meaning and perhaps even a *new normal*, whether or not you ultimately have children or the number of children of which you have dreamed.

I end this book with this chapter in order to help you build on the tools you have acquired to solidify the new normal and find meaning in your experiences. I discuss ways to commemorate your unborn child so that you can honor and cherish the memory of your lost child in a way that facilitates a sense of peace and meaning. I help you to examine the manner in which the reproductive loss might have shaken up your belief system and ways you can incorporate that experience in a healthy way as you redefine your beliefs. I also encourage you to evaluate and, if necessary, redefine your life priorities so that you can live a valued life with grace and dignity, accepting the reproductive loss and achieving quality of life. In the context of the balanced, healthy belief system to which you are shifting, you can create a personal mission statement to guide the choices that you make in any one moment in your life as you work toward achieving your new goals and priorities. I also include a brief section on relapse prevention, which allows you to identify warning signs for the occurrence or reoccurrence of symptoms of depression, anxiety, or other unhealthy ways of coping, and identify ways to address those symptoms. I end the chapter with a brief reflection on finding meaning and cultivating wisdom from the experience of your reproductive loss.

COMMEMORATING YOUR CHILD

Many people who have lost an unborn child or whose newborn lived only a short period of time find a great deal of meaning in commemorating their child, either by permanently displaying a reminder of the baby or by performing a ritual on the anniversary of the loss. Such a remembrance is a time for reflection on your connection with your child, as well as on the manner in which the child touched the lives of you and your family, the manner in which the child brought you and your partner or family together, and the manner in which you achieved personal growth and wisdom. If your remembrance is a special event, it will undoubtedly be a time of tears. However, over time, it is my hope that you can steal some moments of joy or peace as you consider how you made meaning from the experience.

Exhibit 10.1 is a list of ways you might consider commemorating the memory of your child. I cannot take credit for any of these suggestions. They come from other resources on pregnancy loss, the creativity of my own clients who have experienced a pregnancy loss, and stories that I have read of others who have experienced similar tragedies. You might choose one of these on the list, or you might do

---

EXHIBIT 10.1. Commemorating Your Child

- Go to a favorite location (e.g., beach) and spread flower petals or release butterflies.
- Frame a picture of the ultrasound or newborn.
- Wear a necklace with the initials of your baby's name.
- Display a wood carving or some other artistic expression with the initials of your baby's name.
- Read a scripture from the Bible or another holy book.
- Donate flowers to be used in a religious service on or near the anniversary of the loss.
- Light a candle on special dates that you want to remember your baby.
- Plant a tree, bush, or flower in memory of your child.
- Donate to a charity in your baby's name.
- Participate in a walk or run for charity in your baby's name.
- Host a small gathering of close friends and family on the anniversary of the loss or on the baby's due date or birthday.

Note. Please see the following website for additional ideas: http://www.bethmorey.com/p/freebies.html

---

something entirely different. The choice is yours. There is no right or wrong way to commemorate your child. And if you choose not to do anything to commemorate your child, that's OK, too.

SHIFTING YOUR BELIEFS

In Chapters 4 and 5, we considered the types of thoughts that you might experience when you encounter a reminder of your reproductive loss or when you are faced with uncertainty about your reproductive future. Cognitive behavioral therapists call these thoughts *automatic thoughts* because they arise so quickly in any one situation that we often don't realize that they are exerting a profound effect on our mood.

Although these situational automatic thoughts are the ones that cognitive behavioral therapists most frequently work with in treatment, people also are characterized by deeper layers of cognition (i.e., beliefs) that affect the types of thoughts that arise in any one situation. These deeper beliefs are influenced by our formative experiences. Many of these formative experiences occur in childhood, such as when we receive direct or indirect messages from our parents, siblings, teachers, and peers that shape how we view ourselves, other people, the world around us, and the future. However, I have seen time and again that our deeper beliefs are also shaped by defining experiences in adulthood. A reproductive loss would be one of those experiences.

Take some time to think about how your reproductive loss affected your own personal belief system. How do you view yourself? Other people? The world and the future? Have your views in any of these domains fundamentally changed relative to the views in these domains that you had before the loss? Exhibit 10.2 lists examples of beliefs in several domains that might have shifted in a negative direction after your reproductive loss. Do any of these resonate with you? People who have struggled with depression or anxiety might that some of these beliefs were present even before the reproductive loss. Others might have had a relatively positive set of beliefs, only to have them upended after experiencing the reproductive loss.

When negative beliefs such as the ones displayed in Exhibit 10.2 are activated, the likelihood increases that you will experience negative automatic thoughts in specific situations in which you are reminded of the reproductive loss or called on to solve a problem that involves your reproductive future. These beliefs might even increase the likelihood that you experience negative automatic thoughts when you are faced with nonreproductive stressors, such as difficulties on the job or a tense conversation with a friend or family member. As you saw in Chapters 4 and 5, unhelpful automatic thoughts are often

EXHIBIT 10.2. Examples of Unhelpful Beliefs Following a Reproductive Loss

Beliefs About the Self
- I'm incompetent.
- I'm not good enough.
- I'm less than other women (or men).
- I'm undeserving.
- I'm a failure.
- I'm helpless.
- I'm powerless.

Beliefs About Others
- Doctors (or medical staff) are incompetent.
- Doctors (or medical staff) are more concerned about covering their tracks than giving good medical care.
- Everyone else has it easy.
- Everyone else is more deserving than I am.
- Nobody understands.
- Nobody cares.

Beliefs About the World
- The world is cruel.
- The world is dangerous or threatening.

Beliefs About the Future
- Things won't work out.
- I'll never be happy.
- My life will be meaningless.
- I'll be all alone.

associated with a negative shift in mood, which makes you vulnerable to symptoms of depression, anxiety, and anger. Fortunately, the skills you learned in Chapters 4 and 5 will be invaluable in allowing you to catch these automatic thoughts when they arise, critically evaluate their accuracy and usefulness, and develop adaptive responses if you decide there is a more balanced way of viewing these situations.

Although it is helpful, and I would say essential, to have those thought modification skills in place, many cognitive behavioral therapists believe that the most lasting change occurs when a person has shifted away from a set of negative, unhelpful beliefs to a set of beliefs that are more helpful, balanced, and healthy. Such a shift would decrease the likelihood that you will experience negative automatic thoughts in stressful and challenging situations in the first place. The shift does not have to be a dramatic one—in fact, it is important that you identify helpful, balanced, and healthy beliefs that are compelling and believable. For example, if the belief "I'm incompetent" resonated with you, perhaps you work toward adopting a belief such as "I'm just as competent as other people." If the belief "I'll never be happy" resonated with you, perhaps you work toward adopting the belief "Like other people, I will have good times, and I will have bad times." When a more helpful, balanced, and healthy belief system is in place, you will be better able to weather adversity, solve problems, accept compliments, and mindfully acknowledge joys and pleasures than when a more negative belief system is in place.

How does one go about shifting to a more helpful, balanced, and healthy set of beliefs? It's understandable that this might seem like a formidable task in light of the tragedy you have endured. Keep in mind that the shifting of beliefs does not happen overnight, even if they might have seemingly shifted in a negative direction in the single instance in which you experienced your reproductive loss.

The following are some steps that you can follow to work with the beliefs that may be maintaining your emotional distress.

1. Clearly identify one or more unhelpful beliefs about yourself, other people, the world, or the future that can capture the theme that resonates across the negative automatic thoughts that you experience in stressful and challenging situations. It's OK if the items in Exhibit 10.2 don't resonate with you. To identify your own unique beliefs, try keeping a thought record (described in Chapter 4) so that you can prospectively track thoughts that might reflect an underlying theme. Another strategy is to ask, "When I am faced with a stressful or challenging situation, what does this mean to me? What does this mean about me? about others? the world? the future?" Answers to these questions about the meaning of events you experience in your life often give you a clue about the belief that underlies the thoughts that you experience in any one situation.

2. Clearly define the new, more helpful, balanced, and healthy beliefs for which you are striving. Remember to make the new belief balanced and accurate. If it is too positive (e.g., "Life is and will always be great"), then you run the risk of not embracing it as fully as you might if it was more believable.

3. List the new, more helpful, balanced, and healthy belief on a sheet of paper such as the one in Figure 10.1. Then, think back across the course of your life and jot down previous experiences, events, accomplishments, and so on that support the new belief.

4. Keep this sheet of paper handy in the ensuing weeks. Whenever you have an experience, event, or accomplishment that supports the new belief, write it down, no matter how small or insignificant it might seem.

FIGURE 10.1. Evidence Log

Old belief: _____

New belief: _____

Evidence That Supports My New Belief

_____   _____

_____   _____

_____   _____

_____   _____

_____   _____

_____   _____

_____   _____

_____   _____

_____   _____

_____   _____

_____   _____

_____   _____

_____   _____

_____   _____

Circle the degree to which I believe the new belief (in pencil):

0%   10%   20%   30%   40%   50%   60%   70%   80%   90%   100%

5. Each time you write something on the sheet of paper, read through the totality of evidence that supports the new belief and, at the bottom of the page, circle the degree to which you believe the new belief. Notice that I have suggested that you use pencil to circle your rating; this is so because I'd like you to rate the degree to which you believe the new belief *each time* you list evidence, which means you'll be making many ratings. Over time, as evidence accumulates, it is expected that you will believe the new belief to a greater degree. Hence, your ratings will change, so it might be helpful to erase your previous ratings so that the newest rating stands out.

The keys to this and other belief modification exercises are to (a) be realistic and balanced in defining the new belief, (b) ensure that you do not dismiss evidence that supports the new belief, and (c) stick with the process over time because belief modification is a gradual process. Although it is true that many people's beliefs change after a reproductive loss, my wish for you is that, as life goes on, you approach the future with balance and gratitude rather than with pessimism and despair. Your belief system will guide the approach you take. It can become your new normal.

REDEFINING PRIORITIES AND GOALS

Some people find that a tragedy such as a reproductive loss prompts them to examine and redefine their priorities and goals in life. It is understandable that, at the moment, you might be consumed with the goal of getting pregnant again or adding to your family in a different way. It might seem like you do not have the time, energy, or resources to focus on anything else. No one would ever begrudge you of that goal.

However, I'd encourage you to be mindful of the pie chart that was described in Chapter 3. Recall that each piece of the pie represents an important part of your identity or an important pursuit that gives meaning to your life. Together, they represent your value-driven life. If the slice of the pie that represents having a child is not intact, you will have other slices of the pie to carry you through, giving you meaning and purpose. If you ultimately have fewer children than you had hoped to have, you will play many other valued roles that will contribute to your living a valued life. Your priorities and goals will be enriching and varied.

As much as is possible, I'd encourage you to start or continue to do things that fall into as many slices of your pie chart as possible. Doing so will help you to bear any further bumps in the road that you may experience with your reproductive health or journey to completing your family. If you're currently engaging in time-consuming activities such as ongoing fertility treatment or adoption, this might be impossible. However, you can nevertheless reflect on your priorities and goals, defining your ideal slices of pie and envisioning the manner in which you might pursue them when you are ready.

The bottom line is this: You will be able to live a joyful, valued, meaningful life with grace, dignity, and gratitude regardless of the number of children in your household. It might not seem like it right now, but it will happen. The way to do it is to think broadly, beyond your reproductive loss and struggles, to define those goals and priorities and, when you are ready, move forward in a way that embraces them.

YOUR PERSONAL MISSION STATEMENT

What I have discussed in this chapter so far—adopting a balanced and healthy belief system, creating a vision of your priorities and goals in the context of a valued life, and then enacting that vision—

might seem like too much. These goals are, admittedly, quite lofty, but for my clients and I, they helped us to be mindful of the "big picture," and it gave us hope that although life might seem hopeless and empty at the moment, we were not predestined to live a life of hopelessness and emptiness forever. In each moment, you have a choice. You can choose to act according to despair over what you don't have. Or to can choose to act according to your strengths, your values, and what you do have. There will undoubtedly be moments in which the former wins out. You're only human. When the latter wins out, you will be taking a step toward living a life with grace and dignity.

Many of my clients find it helpful to develop a personal mission statement that guides the way they view and respond to a situation in any one moment. Thus, even if you are caught up in a moment of intense emotion and can't remember your values, or you can't remember the tools that you've acquired by reading this book, a simple mission statement can help you to stop and think about whether you are moving toward the person you want to be or moving away from the person you want to be.

The mission statement can take many forms, depending on what you would find most helpful. For example, it can be a statement that summarizes your most salient strengths. Amelia created such a statement: "I am a person who is balanced and connected with others." When she found herself in moments of emotional upset, when she wanted to isolate herself from others or give up, she repeated this statement to herself and asked herself, "Am I responding in a manner that promotes balance and connection with others?" If the answer was no, she asked herself, "How can I better respond in a way that builds on my strengths of being balanced and connected with others?"

Another version of the mission statement can emphasize a particular value or set of values that by which you want to live. Angela, for example, valued and found great meaning in her connection with nature. She loved taking daytrips to locations with beautiful scenery, and she enjoyed activities such as hiking, biking, and kayaking. Whenever she opted not to engage in these sorts of activities, she knew she was "off." She composed the mission statement "The wonder of nature heals all wounds." When she found herself in moments of emotional upset, she repeated this statement to herself and asked herself, "Am I responding in a manner that is consistent with my belief about my connection with nature? Or am I ignoring a powerful healing force in my life?"

You can also develop a mission statement on the basis of the wisdom that you have gained in psychotherapy or in reading a self-help book such as this one. Jill, for example, developed this mission statement: "Above all, I want to live a rich, valued life." When she noticed herself avoiding engagement in her life, she asked herself, "Will this decision help me to live a rich, valued life?"

A fourth approach to developing a mission statement is to develop a decision tree that can guide the choices you make in particular situations. Karen, for example, knew that she got meaning from helping others but also struggled with assertiveness and had a tendency to take on more than she could handle, leaving little time for self-care. As she was in the midst of the adoption process after two rounds of unsuccessful IVF, she knew that she needed to approach the things she took on her life with a balance between acting according to her value of serving others and taking care of herself. She developed a two-pronged decision tree: "(1) Am I saying yes to this person because it is truly consistent with my value of serving others? and (2) Will saying yes have a negative effect on my own well-being?" If she answered yes to the first question and no to the second question, she would then say yes to whatever request was being made of her. However, if the request did not meet these two criteria, then she used the communication skills described in Chapter 6 to politely decline the request.

A final approach to developing a mission statement is to have some sort of a role model in mind that you can envision when you are deciding on a particular course of action. Such a role model would encapsulate the characteristics, strengths, and values that you are working toward integrating into your own life. It could be a public figure. Some of my clients have looked to a public figure like Bethany Hamilton, the surfer who lost her arm in a shark attack and who continued to pursue her dreams and live a life of faith and optimism. Other people look to people they know in their own lives who exemplify valued strengths and characteristics or to people who have touched their lives in some way. Kristin remembered early in her pregnancy before her loss that a friend of the family brought her a small gift for her unborn child. That family friend had been struggling with a number of unsuccessful trials of IVF. Kristin remembered being quite moved by the fact that this family friend was genuinely happy for her and expressed a great deal of kindness despite her own reproductive struggles. She decided that this was the type of person that she wanted to be following her own loss and that doing so would help her own healing.

Mission statements need not be limited to these examples. Indeed, there are entire courses on the development of personal mission statements offered in settings as diverse as business schools and places of worship that can guide you in developing rich and nuanced mission statements that touch on multiple aspects of your strengths and values. If you are a person who would thrive on such an undertaking, by all means, pursue that avenue. It is likely that doing so will help you to achieve many of the aims described in this chapter, including shaping a healthy belief system, redefining goals and priorities, and living a valued life. However, that might be too overwhelming for you right now. Having a simple statement, or a simple decision tree, or an image of a person who encompasses the person you strive to be, might be most accessible in times of emotional upset and struggle.

RELAPSE PREVENTION

Relapse prevention is a strategy that helps people avoid a relapse or a recurrence of substantial emotional distress in the future. This is not to say that you will never again experience emotional upset at a reminder of your reproductive loss. Occasional tearfulness, sadness, longing, anger, frustration, and envy are to be expected. When I say *substantial emotional distress*, I'm referring to emotional upset that causes problems in your life, such as not taking care of yourself, difficulty completing tasks at work or home, tension in relationships with others, or emotional upset that is significant enough that others notice and express concern about you.

It's helpful to have a plan in place for dealing with an exacerbation of emotional distress. Often, when people are in the throes of emotional distress, it's difficult to remember what they have learned in the past to manage it. Having a game plan on a single sheet of paper will serve as a concrete reminder that you can manage emotional distress and will recap how to do it. You can use Figure 10.2 to develop your own personalized plan.

The relapse prevention plan has five components. First, it is helpful to recognize the *warning signs* that the relapse prevention plan is needed in the first place. It is important to be aware of these warning signs because, all too often, we go about living our lives without noticing subtle indicators that something is "off" (i.e., living in automatic pilot mode), and before we know it, we are overcome by another episode of emotional distress. Warning signs can mean different things to different people. Sometimes warning signs are a noticeable increase in an undesirable emotional state, such as depression, sadness, anxiety, or anger. Sometimes warning signs could be an increase in the frequency of unhelpful thoughts, for example, "Things won't get better" or "I'm a failure." In other instances, warning signs can be things that you are doing that you know are not healthy, such

FIGURE 10.2. Relapse Prevention Plan

My Relapse Prevention Plan
Warning signs:
Tools I can use to cope:
People I can contact for support:
How I will know if I need professional help:
Names of professionals I can contact:

as an increase in using alcohol or drugs, overeating, staying up all night, or isolating yourself. Warning signs can also take the form of comments made and concerns expressed by others.

The second section of the relapse prevention plan allows you to summarize the coping tools that have worked best for you in the past in managing emotional upset. Many of the tools you jot down may have been described in this book, but they certainly don't have to be limited to those. Be thoughtful about the coping tools that might need additional description. For example, you might have found thought modification to be helpful. However, in the midst of another episode of emotional upset, you might forget the steps to achieve thought modification. Thus, it might be helpful to record additional reminders, such as ways to question unhelpful thoughts (e.g., "What evidence supports and refutes this thought? What would I tell a friend in this situation?").

In the third section of the relapse prevention plan, you will write down the names of people whom you can contact for support. Be sure there is more than one name on this list. Also be sure to record each person's contact information (e.g., cell phone number, land-line number, e-mail address). These days, most of us no longer memorize telephone numbers because they are easily stored in our list of contacts. However, trust me when I say there may come a time when you need to contact someone but your phone will be out of power, and you won't be able to access his or her contact information. Having this information written down averts dependence on technology.

In many instances, the first three steps of the relapse prevention plan will be sufficient. You will notice the warning signs, and you will be able to gather yourself in such a way that you implement your coping tools and utilize your social support network. Although you might never need them, it is important to plan for instances when professional help is warranted. Go back to Chapter 1 if you need a reminder of the guidelines I presented to determine when professional help is warranted. One rule of thumb is that the emotional state you are experiencing or the choices you make are putting yourself or others at risk, then it is important to seek professional help. However, this is certainly not the only rule of thumb, and it will be important for you to identify, in advance, unique signals for you that professional help would be indicated. In the last section of the relapse prevention plan, write the names and phone numbers of some professionals you might contact. These might include a previous therapist or psychiatrist, or they might include other trusted health care professionals (e.g., your primary care physician, your gynecologist, your fertility doctor). However, you can also provide some names of mental health professionals with whom you have not met but who practice in a convenient location and who might accept your insurance plan. Again, you might never need this information, but if you do, doing the legwork now to compile it will help you to feel less overwhelmed and more ready to take action if appropriate.

After you complete the relapse prevention plan, think of where you will keep it. You will want to have easy access to it if it is needed. Perhaps you tuck it away inside of this book. Perhaps you have a folder where you have compiled a number of the activities that you completed while you read this book. The relapse prevention plan will only be effective to the degree that you can find it and use it.

FINDING MEANING

A common and natural response to reproductive loss and trauma is "Why do bad things happen to good people?" It is so difficult to make sense of the loss of a child. One would never, ever suggest that you look for the "good" or the "silver lining." It's tragic any way you look at it.

When I think about finding meaning from reproductive loss and trauma, I think back to research conducted by Dr. Heidi Stiegelis and her colleagues in The Netherlands. They asked patients with cancer and healthy members of a control group who did not have cancer to complete a number of self-report inventories assessing aspects of positive functioning. The researchers found that on three occasions across radiation treatment and a 3-month follow-up period, cancer patients reported *higher* levels of optimism and self-esteem. How could that be? Were the cancer patients in denial about the severity of their illness? Not at all. My explanation is that the cancer patients had learned to savor each moment they had, expressing gratitude for all that they had experienced in their lives, acknowledging their strengths, forgiving the transgressions of others, and not dwelling on negative things that were out of their control. They had found meaning. Despite having a serious illness, they were living life on their own terms.

That is the task for all of us who have experienced a reproductive loss or trauma. For those of us who go on to have a child, that "victory" will taste all the sweeter given our unfortunate histories. For those of us who have little ones in the extended family, we will nurture those relationships and create special bonds that will last a lifetime. For those of us who decide to reach out and help others who have experienced similar losses, we know that our unborn or deceased child will be making a positive and lasting impact in this world. For those of us who are people of faith, we might foster an intimate relationship with God or become more deeply involved in spiritual practice.

Regardless of whether you decide to adopt a child, forge relationships with nieces and nephews, help others who have experienced similar losses, develop a closer relationship with God, or do something else, there is meaning to be had. Living a valued life according to your strengths, savoring the small moments of pleasure or gratitude, and embracing each moment in a mindful, nonjudgmental manner will help you to attain a sense of peace that will provide meaning and connection with others. Along the way of your journey to this peace, you will develop insight and wisdom that you had not thought were possible to achieve. The journey is an emotional one, and it might seem like you're not sure which direction you're moving in at any one moment. The journey does not necessarily end. And though you did not choose to go on this journey, you can choose to embrace it with grace and dignity. You will become a stronger, more empathetic person because of it. You will demonstrate resilience. My sincerest best wishes to you, the reader, as you forge your own unique journey toward a fulfilling, valued life.

POSTSCRIPT

I struggled with the decision of whether or not to share whether I have any children. After all, a major premise of my book is that life can be meaningful *with or without children*, and I observed several times throughout the book that it can be difficult for people who have experienced reproductive loss without children to believe that authors of books such as this can understand their experience if the authors do indeed have children.

I decided that readers deserve to know, both out of the profound respect I have for people who read this book as well as to give a sense of optimism and hope for the future.

I lost my son in March 2009. Over the course of several months, my grief subsided and I reengaged with the world, but I was uncertain that I would have children due to advanced maternal age and the lack of explanation for the cause of my loss. I had a great deal of difficulty being around other women my age who had young children. In December 2009, after several months of trying, I learned that I was pregnant again. From 18 to 36 weeks' gestation, I was given weekly progesterone shots to prevent preterm labor. I experienced a great deal of anxiety about losing this child and tried to avoid, as much as possible, telling others that I was pregnant. Throughout the pregnancy, I applied the cognitive behavioral strategies described in this book over and over and over again, just as I had after losing the first pregnancy.

I ultimately carried my daughter past full-term—to the point that she was so large that she had difficulty getting through the birth canal and required an emergency cesarean section. She was born on August 10, 2010, when I was 38 years old, weighing 9 pounds and 12 ounces. She was a healthy, alert baby who has turned into a happy, well-adjusted toddler. I'd like to be able to give her a younger sibling, particularly in light of the fact that she has been anointed the "baby whisperer" by the teachers at her school because she is so good with the little ones. But it does not look like that is in the cards for us. It's OK. We're focused on the many advantages that we can give a single child. Thus, I'm continuing my pursuit of a life well lived, as a parent as well as by cultivating and trying to thrive in many, many other areas of my life and taking care to acknowledge the many benefits of raising a single child in a close-knit household with my husband.

I should contrast my story, though, with that of a close friend of mine. In her late 30s, she and her husband went through a couple of rounds of IVF. They were unsuccessful, and rather than continuing to try, she decided to pursue a different dream—she went back to graduate school to get her PhD. She obtained her degree and currently holds her "dream job," where every day she sees how her work is making a tangible difference in people's lives. She and her husband fill their evenings and weekends to the brim, engaging in activities that they find joyful and meaningful. In fact, the two of them modified their home to accommodate pursuits about which each one is passionate—she has a full home gym and a sauna; her husband has a full music studio. She and her husband have an extraordinary connection and authentic respect and admiration for one another. She is the happiest, most well-adjusted person I have ever met, and she undoubtedly meets the criteria for a "life well lived."

Regardless of whether you ultimately have children, my wish for you is that you live mindfully according to your values, accepting moments of emotional upset and keeping them in perspective. There are many roads to resilience and happiness. I encourage you to begin paving your own road with grace and dignity.

APPENDIX:
MINDFULNESS RESOURCES

BOOKS

Brantley, J. (2007). *Calming your anxious mind: How mindfulness & compassion can free you from anxiety, fear, and panic* (2nd ed.). Oakland, CA: New Harbinger.

Hanh, T. N. (1976). *The miracle of mindfulness: An introduction to the practice of meditation.* Boston, MA: Beacon Press.

Hanh, T. N. (2011). *Peace is every breath: A practice for our busy lives.* New York, NY: HarperOne.

Kabat-Zinn, J. (1990). *Full catastrophe living.* New York, NY: Bantam Dell.

Kabat-Zinn, J. (1994). *Wherever you go, there you are.* New York, NY: Hyperion.

Kabat-Zinn, J. (2005). *Coming to our senses: Healing ourselves and the world through mindfulness.* New York, NY: Hyperion.

Kabat-Zinn, J. (2012). *Mindfulness for beginners: Reclaiming the present moment—and your life.* Boulder, CO: Sounds True. (CD included)

Orsillo, S. M., & Roemer, L. (2011). *The mindful way through anxiety: Break free from chronic worry and reclaim your life.* New York, NY: Guilford Press. (Mindfulness exercises can be found at http://mindful waythroughanxietybook.com)

Stahl, B., & Goldstein, E. (2010). *A mindfulness-based stress reduction workbook.* Oakland, CA: New Harbinger. (CD included)

Tirch, D. D. (2012). *The compassionate mind guide to overcoming anxiety: Using compassion-focused therapy to calm worry, panic, and fear.* Oakland, CA: New Harbinger Publications. (Mindfulness exercises can be found at http://www.mindfulcompassion.com/cms)

Williams, M., & Penman, D. (2011). *Mindfulness: An eight-week plan for finding peace in a frantic world.* New York, NY: Rodale. (Mindfulness exercises can be found at http://franticworld.com)

Williams, M., Teasdale, J., Segal, Z., & Kabat-Zinn, J. (2007). *The mindful way through depression: Freeing yourself from chronic unhappiness.* New York, NY: Guilford Press. (CD included)

CDs

Brach, T. (2012). *Mindfulness meditation: Nine guided practices to awaken presence and open your heart.* Boulder, CO: Sounds True.

Kabat-Zinn, J. (2002). *Guided mindfulness meditation: Series 1.* Boulder, CO: Sounds True.

Kabat-Zinn, J. (2012). *Guided mindfulness meditation: Series 3.* Boulder, CO: Sounds True.

NOTES

INTRODUCTION

Jaffe, J., & Diamond, M. O. (2011). *Reproductive trauma: Psychotherapy with infertility and pregnancy loss clients.* Washington, DC: American Psychological Association. doi:10.1037/12347-000

CHAPTER I

Bonanno, G. A., Westphal, M., & Mancini, A. D. (2011). Resilience to loss and potential trauma. *Annual Review of Clinical Psychology, 7,* 511–535. doi:10.1146/annurev-clinpsy-032210-104526

Malkinson, R. (2007). *Cognitive grief therapy: Constructing a rational meaning to life following loss.* New York, NY: Norton.

Meert, K. L., Shear, K., Newth, C. J. L., Harrison, R., Berger, J., Zimmerman, J., . . . Eunice Kennedy Shriver National Institute of Public Health and Human Development Collaborative Pediatric Critical Care Research Network. (2011). Follow-up study of complicated grief among parents eighteen months after a child's death in the pediatric intensive care unit. *Journal of Palliative Medicine, 14,* 207–214. doi:10.1089/jpm.2010.0291

Shear, M. K., & Mulhare, E. (2008). Complicated grief. *Psychiatric Annals, 38,* 663–670. doi:10.3928/00485713-20081001-10

CHAPTER 2

Hauri, P., & Linde, S. (1996). *No more sleepless nights* (Revised edition). New York, NY: Wiley.

Lewinsohn, P. M., Sullivan, J. M., & Grosscup, S. J. (1980). Changing reinforcing events: An approach to the treatment of depression. *Psychotherapy: Theory, Research, & Practice, 17,* 322–334. doi:10.1037/h0085929

Linehan, M. M. (1993). *Skills training manual for borderline personality disorder.* New York, NY: Guilford Press.

McKay, M., Wood, J. C., & Brantley, J. (2007). *The dialectical behavior therapy skills workbook: Practical DBT exercises for learning mindfulness, interpersonal effectiveness, emotion regulation, & distress tolerance.* Oakland, CA: New Harbinger.

Otto, M. W., & Smits, J. A. J. (2011). *Exercise for mood and anxiety: Proven strategies for overcoming depression and enhancing wellbeing.* New York, NY: Oxford University Press.

Perlis, M. L., Jungquist, C., Smith, M. T., & Posner, D. (2005). *Cognitive behavioral treatment of insomnia: A session-by-session guide.* New York, NY: Springer-Verlag.

Silberman, S. A. (2008). *The insomnia workbook.* Oakland, CA: New Harbinger.

Smits, J. A. J., & Otto, M. W. (2009). *Exercise for mood and anxiety disorders: Therapist guide* (Treatments That Work series). New York, NY: Oxford University Press.

Wegner, D. (1989). *White bears and other unwanted thoughts: Suppression, obsession, and the psychology of mental control.* New York, NY: Penguin Press.

CHAPTER 3

Dimidjian, S., Barrera, M., Jr., Martell, C., Muñoz, R. F., & Lewinsohn, P. M. (2011). The origins and current status of behavioral activation treatments for depression. *Annual Review of Clinical Psychology, 7,* 1–38. doi:10.1146/annurev-clinpsy-032210-104535

Dimidjian, S., Hollon, S. D., Dobson, K. S., Schmaling, K. B., Kohlenberg, R. J., Addis, M. E., . . . Jacobson, N. S. (2006). Randomized trial of behavioral activation, cognitive therapy, and antidepressant medication in the acute treatment of adults with major depression. *Journal of Consulting and Clinical Psychology, 74,* 658–670. doi:10.1037/0022-006X.74.4.658

CHAPTER 4

Rothbaum, B. O., Foa, E. B., & Hembree, E. A. (2007). *Reclaiming your life from a traumatic experience: Workbook.* New York, NY: Oxford University Press.

CHAPTER 5

Dugas, M. J., Gagnon, F., Ladouceur, R., & Freeston, M. H. (1998). Generalized anxiety disorder: Preliminary test of a conceptual model. *Behaviour Research and Therapy, 36,* 215–226. doi:10.1016/S0005-7967(97)00070-3

CHAPTER 6

Gottman, J. (1994). *Why marriages succeed or fail . . . and how you can make yours last.* New York, NY: Simon & Schuster.

Greil, A. L., Schmidt, L., & Peterson, B. D. (2014). Perinatal experiences associated with infertility. In A. Wenzel & S. Stuart (Eds.), *Oxford handbook of perinatal psychology.* New York, NY: Oxford University Press.

Newman, S. (2011). *The case for the only child: Your essential guide.* Deerfield Beach, FL: Health Communications.

CHAPTER 7

Abramowitz, J. S., Deacon, B. J., & Whiteside, S. P. H. (2011). *Exposure therapy for anxiety: Principles and practice.* New York, NY: Guilford Press.

Craske, M. G., Kircanski, K., Zeilowsky, M., Mystkowski, J., Chowdhury, N., & Baker, A. (2008). Optimizing inhibitory learning during exposure therapy. *Behaviour Research and Therapy, 46*, 5–27.

Lang, A. J., & Craske, M. G. (2000). Manipulations of exposure-based therapy to reduce return of fear: A replication. *Behaviour Research and Therapy, 38*, 1–12. doi:10.1016/S0005-7967(99)00031-5

CHAPTER 8

D'Zurilla, T. J., & Nezu, A. M. (2007). *Problem-solving therapy: A positive approach to clinical intervention* (3rd ed.). New York, NY: Springer.

CHAPTER 9

Kabat-Zinn, J. (1994). *Wherever you go there you are.* New York, NY: Hyperion.

Kleiman, K. K. (2009). *Therapy and the postpartum woman: Notes on healing postpartum depression for clinicians and the women who seek their help.* New York, NY: Routledge.

Linehan, M. M. (1993). *Skills training manual for borderline personality disorder.* New York, NY: Guilford Press.

Segal, Z. V., Williams, J. M. G., & Teasdale, J. D. (2013). *Mindfulness-based cognitive therapy for depression* (2nd ed.). New York, NY: Guilford Press.

CHAPTER 10

Stiegleis, H. E., Hagedoorn, M., Sanderman, R., van der Zee, K. I., Buunk, B. P., & van den Bergh, A. C. M. (2003). Cognitive adaptation: A comparison of cancer patients and healthy references. *British Journal of Health Psychology, 8*, 303–318. doi:10.1348/135910703322370879

INDEX

ABOUT THE AUTHOR

Amy Wenzel, PhD, is owner of Wenzel Consulting, LLC, clinical assistant professor at the University of Pennsylvania School of Medicine, adjunct faculty at the Beck Institute for Cognitive Behavior Therapy, and affiliate at the Postpartum Stress Center. She is the author or editor of 14 books and approximately 100 peer-reviewed journal articles and book chapters, many on the topic of cognitive behavioral therapy and perinatal psychology. She lectures internationally on these topics and regularly provides workshops and webinars to clinicians who are acquiring skill in CBT. Her research has been funded by the National Institute of Mental Health, the American Foundation for Suicide Prevention, and the National Alliance for Research on Schizophrenia and Depression (now the Brain and Behavior Foundation). She currently divides her time between scholarly writing and research, training and consultation, and clinical practice. A full description of Dr. Wenzel's professional activities can be found at http://dramywenzel.com.

10/15　θ　(10/14)
6/17　①　11/15